ASHP's **Management PEARLS**

Deborah Swartwood Ash, MS

President and CEO
Ash Pharmacy Consultants
Jacksonville, Florida

American Society of Health-System Pharmacists®
Bethesda, MD

Any correspondence regarding this publication should be sent to the publisher, American Society of Health-System Pharmacists, 7272 Wisconsin Avenue, Bethesda, MD 20814, attention: Special Publishing.

Director, Special Publishing: Jack Bruggeman

Senior Editorial Project Manager: Dana Battaglia

Page Design: Carol Barrer

Library of Congress Cataloging-in-Publication Data

ASHP's management pearls / [edited by] Deborah Swartwood Ash.

p. ; cm.

Includes bibliographical references and index.

ISBN 978-1-58528-219-7

1. Pharmacy management--Congresses. I. Ash, Deborah Swartwood. II. American Society of Health-System Pharmacists. III. ASHP Midyear Clinical Meeting (42nd : 2007 : Las Vegas, Nev.) IV. Title: Management pearls. V. Title: American Society of Health-System Pharmacists' management pearls.

[DNLM: 1. Pharmacy Service, Hospital--organization & administration--Congresses. 2. Drug Therapy--Congresses. WX 179 A8267 2008]

RS100.A74 2008

615'.1068--dc22

2008038686

ISBN: 978-1-58528-219-7

Contents

Part 1: Personnel Development and Management

Part 2: Program Development, Implementation, and Management

Part 3: Financial Management

Note from the Publisher

The Pearls sessions at the ASHP Midyear Clinical Meeting (MCM) are some of the best-attended sessions each year. With the publication of the "Pearls" series, ASHP is attempting to capture the best of these presentations with more in-depth coverage, which is not possible under the strict time constraints of the MCM pearls presentations. We hope you find this compilation worthwhile.

We encourage ASHP members to participate in the MCM Pearls presentations. To those who are participating in upcoming Pearl sessions, we hope you will consider turning those presentations into chapters for the Pearls book series. For additional information on becoming a Pearls series author, please contact me at jbruggeman@ashp.org

Preface

In this era of limited resources, complex evolving regulation, constantly changing technology and accreditation standards, and rising drug costs, how do pharmacy managers successfully maneuver the maze and insure that patients receive optimal medication therapy at an acceptable cost to their healthcare systems?

It is difficult to excel as both a pharmacist clinician and pharmacy manager. Pharmacy directors and managers are trained first as pharmacists and then in the area of management. This management training may either be formal, such as in graduate programs and residencies, or informal, primarily through mentorship. Pharmacy management is a significant challenge in small hospitals, where managers by necessity must be competent in both the role of clinician and manager. It is a challenge in larger health systems as well, as organizations flatten their management levels. Pharmacy management, while similar to other businesses, also adds the complexity of State and Federal Pharmacy Regulations, JCAHO and possibly NCQA accreditation, and OSHA and other hazardous materials regulations. Therefore, obtaining and maintaining competencies to be an effective pharmacy manager and leader continues to challenge the profession.

In the US, economic leadership is shifting from energy, financials, and materials to health care, telecommunications and consumer staples, according to Richard Bernstein, Chief Investment Strategist, Merrill Lynch.[1] This shift to health care will increase the current burden on pharmacy management to meet their financial targets. Not only will financial pressures increase within the pharmacy manager's organization, but also contractual burdens will escalate with outside companies, such as health insurers and group purchasing organizations. Managing a hospital pharmacy department is comparable to running a stand-alone business. The 2007 ASHP National Survey of Pharmacy Practice in Hospital Settings estimates the average acquisition cost for inpatient pharmaceuticals at $ 5 million with a range from approximately $700,000 to over $17 million, and outpatient pharmaceuticals are estimated to average $3.7 million with a range from approximately $600,000 to over $10 million.[2] Add to this pharmaceutical cost the expenses of technology and personnel and the hospital pharmacy budget is significant in hospitals of all sizes.

The pharmacy department is unique from other hospital departments, in that the majority of operating costs are derived from pharmaceutical inventory and technology as opposed to personnel costs. Therefore, pharmacy directors focus on the larger costs (pharmaceuticals and technology) and accreditation requirements often at the expense of personnel management. Keeping up-to-date with trends and skills in personnel management is formidable but necessary. The 2007 ASHP National Survey of Pharmacy Practice in hospital settings estimates that 6.4% of FTE pharmacists' positions are vacant nationally.[3] In institutions of less than 50 beds or 50 to 99 beds, these vacancies climb to 7.7 % and 9.7 %, respectively.[4] This continuing scarcity of resources makes effective personnel management one of the key attributes for pharmacy directors and managers.

The ASHP Section of Pharmacy Practice Managers instituted the Management Pearls session at the 2005 Clinical Midyear meeting to address the continuing need to provide managerial programs for both new and seasoned pharmacy managers and leaders. The program allows attendees to obtain current strategies from colleagues to improve pharmacy services, implement pharmacy improvements, and share human resource opportunities that have been implemented successfully. These "Pearls" aim to convey in a short period of time a single idea, concept, or fact that may not be widely known, understood, published, or taught. For the pharmacy managers or leaders "stretched thin" or required to wear "two hats," obtaining some Pearls on successful personnel, program, or financial management strategies can be an effective way to close this knowledge gap.

However, for managers with limited travel budgets or personnel vacancies, attending educational programs may not be an option. For others, obtaining additional information, forms, or details from these Pearls presentations is desirable. To meet these additional pharmacy leader needs, ASHP has developed the Management Pearls book. This is a collection of Pearls from the 2007 Management Pearls session in Las Vegas. Authors have expanded the information provided at the Pearls session, included forms and computer screen prints, and shared contact information for those who want more information. A special thank you is extended to these authors, who have taken the additional time in their busy management schedules to share their information with colleagues. In reading these Pearls, if a thought is generated for a new program, improvement of a current program, or different way of managing staff in your department for the further improvement of patient care, this book will be a success.

Deborah Swartwood Ash, MS
President, CEO
Ash Pharmacy Consultants
Jacksonville, Florida
debswart@gmail.com

References

1. Bernstein J. Outlook 2008, A Global Forecast and Investment Opportunities For The Year Ahead. *Merrill Lynch Advisor.* Merrill Lynch, Pierce, Fenner and Smith Incorporated, USA; 2008:8-9.
2. Pedersen CA, Schneider PJ, Scheckelhoff DJ. ASHP National survey of Pharmacy Practice in hospital settings: Prescribing and transcribing – 2007. *Am J Hosp Pharm* 2008;65:838.
3. Pedersen CA, Schneider PJ, Scheckelhoff DJ. ASHP National survey of Pharmacy Practice in hospital settings: Prescribing and transcribing – 2007. *Am J Hosp Pharm* 2008;65:841.
4. Pedersen CA, Schneider PJ, Scheckelhoff DJ. ASHP National survey of Pharmacy Practice in hospital settings: Prescribing and transcribing – 2007. *Am J Hosp Pharm* 2008;65:839

Contributors

Della Abboud, PharmD, MBA
Pharmacy Manager
Barnes-Jewish West County Hospital
Creve Coeur, Missouri
dellaa@juno.com

E. Thomas Carey, PharmD
Director of Pharmacy Services
SwedishAmerican Hospital
Rockford, Illinois
tcarey@swedishamerican.org

Tammy Cohen, BS, PharmD, MS
Director of Pharmacy
Baylor Heart and Vascular Hospital and
System Clinical Director of Pharmacy
Baylor Health Care System
Dallas, Texas
tammyco@baylorhealth.edu

John H. Eastham, PharmD
Medication Safety Specialist
Palomar Pomerado Health
Escondido, California
john.eastham@pph.org

Michael A. Fotis, BSPharm
Manager Drug Information and Drug Use Policy, Residency Program Director
Director Education Affairs ICHP
Northwestern Memorial Hospital
Chicago, Illinois
mfotis@nmh.org

Joel A. Hennenfent, PharmD, MBA, BCPS
Director, Pharmacy Services - Clinical Pharmacy and Data Services
Operations Department, Broadlane
St. Louis, Missouri
joel.hennenfent@broadlane.com

Rachel E. Hroncich, PharmD
Clinical Coordinator
Presbyterian Healthcare Services
Albuquerque, New Mexico
rhroncic@phs.org

Anne T. Jarrett, MS
ATJ Consulting, LLC
High Point, North Carolina
ajarrett@triad.rr.com

Annette M. Karageanes, MS
Clinical Resource Specialist, Pharmacy Services
Ascension Health
Grosse Point Woods, Michigan
akarageanes@ascensionhealth.org

Stanley S. Kent, MS, FASHP
Assistant Vice President
Evanston Northwestern Healthcare
Evanston, Illinois
Skent@enh.org

Kristi K. Killelea, PharmD, BCPS
Clinical Manager
Evanston Northwestern Healthcare
Evanston, Illinois
kkillelea@enh.org

Larry J. Koesterer, BS, Pharm, MBA
Senior Director, Group Purchasing, Support Services
Ascension Health
St. Louis, Missouri
lkoesterer@ascensionhealth.org

Georgeanne S. Lemanowicz, BS, Pharm
Pharmacy Information Specialist
Southwest General Health Center
Middleburg Heights, Ohio
glemanowicz@swgeneral.com

Lisa Michener, PharmD, MS
Pharmacy Manager, Clinical Services
Evanston Northwestern Healthcare
Glenview, Illinois
lmichener@enh.org

Nancy Thai Nguyen, PharmD
Pharmacy Supervisor
Cedars-Sinai Medical Center
Los Angeles, California
Nancy.Nguyen@cshs.org

Erin Sears, Pharm D
Clinical Pharmacist, Drug Information
Baylor University Medical Center
Dallas, Texas
Erinse@baylorhealth.edu

Elizabeth M. Schmitz, PharmD, BCPS
Coordinator of Pharmacy Clinical Services
Children's Mercy Hospital
Kansas City, Missouri
Eschmitz0720@yahoo.com

Rita Shane, PharmD, FASHP
Director, Pharmacy Services
Cedars-Sinai Medical Center
Los Angeles, California
shane@cshs.org

Sara J. White, MS, FASHP
Pharmacy Leadership Coach
Mountain View, California
RxSJW@yahoo.com

Part 1

Personnel Development and Management

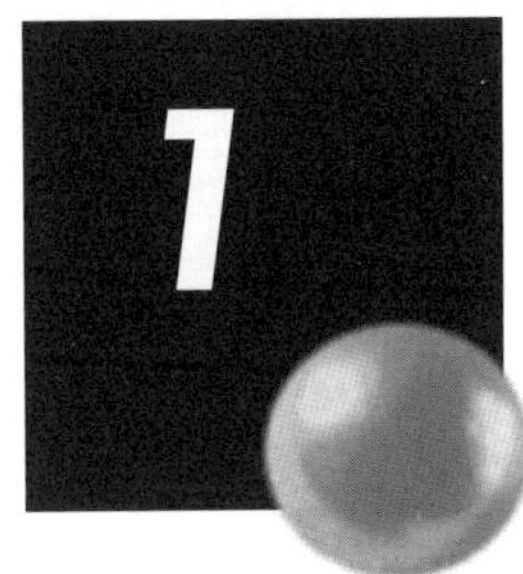

Mentoring: Mentoring for Recruitment and Retention

Sara J. White

Introduction

Pharmacy personnel are faced with many new and expanded roles as the healthcare system rapidly evolves. Some examples of these new roles include pharmacists practicing specifically in the emergency room and anticoagulation clinics, servicing assisted living facilities, and compounding gene therapy. With the implementation of electronic medical records and computerized physician order entry, pharmacy personnel are being needed to assist in the design of these systems, build the medication databases, and develop work processes for not only pharmacy but assist physicians and nurses with their workflow to ensure the continued medication safety in the system. Some traditionally acute clinical practices such as bone marrow transplantation now involve an ambulatory component so pharmacy roles are also expanding.

Not only are pharmacy roles expanding but so is the demand for pharmacy personnel. As the approximately 76 million baby boomers approach retirement, they will increasingly access the healthcare system increasing demand.[1] The continuum of care has also expanded from just the community and hospital pharmacy practice to assisted-living facilities, long-term care, skilled nursing facilities, ambulatory surgery centers, home health agencies, infusion centers, multiple general medicine and specialty ambulatory clinics, sleep clinics, sports clinics, travel clinics, urgent care facilities, emergency rooms, acute care hospitals—all of which use medications and thus need pharmacy services.

Along with pharmacy roles expanding, additional people accessing the healthcare system, more sites that need the pharmacy services, a shortage of pharmacy personnel has developed even in the face of additional new Schools of Pharmacy and technician training programs.[1] These shortages will not be mitigated anytime soon nor will the increasing use of technology offset the need for pharmacy personnel.[1] To maintain and expand pharmacy services, pharmacy departments must be the "employer of choice" in such a competitive labor market. Being the employer of choice means being able not only to recruit new talent but also equally important, retain the current talent. Because each pharmacy employee has many employment options, one approach to being the "employer of choice" is to use mentoring as a strategy for retention and as a carrot for new practitioners choosing where to practice as they transition from school to practice. It is very important to young people that they continue to grow and develop. Mentoring is also a way to develop current talent for these new expanded roles.

Mentoring

The term *mentor* comes from Greek mythology.[2] Homer in the Odyssey has Odysseus choosing Mentor as the guardian for his son Telemachus when he left for the Trojan War.[2] A mentor is defined by Funk and Wagnall's as "a wise and trusted teacher, guide and friend; an elderly monitor or advisor."[3] Coaching and mentoring are sometimes used interchangeably. For our purposes, let's define coaching as helping someone develop certain basic skills, such as how to educate patients, evaluate a therapeutic regimen, or supervise. Mentoring can be thought of as much broader than skill development and include career development, decision options, and self development. For this discussion, coaching is part of mentoring because mentoring should take a holistic approach. Mentoring can provide insights on technical matters, how to interact with others, make decisions, or adapt to a corporate culture or work environment. It also helps the person grow in their capabilities and independence. The success of mentoring depends in large part on the effectiveness of the mentor and the mentoring process.

Characteristics of Successful Mentors and the Mentoring Process

Because a mentor is a trusted advisor who one turns to periodically for career counsel, successful mentors are people who are absolutely credible and whose integrity transcends their message whether it is positive or negative. Mentors are never trying to manipulate but rather have the protégé's best interest in mind. Mentors are authentic individuals who have the time, expertise, and interest in mentoring. A mentor has to be willing to offer knowledge, insights, and wisdom. A mentor needs also to be willing to have an extended relationship with the protégé so they can assist in that person's self discovery. This self discovery entails what really matters, such as what kind of work they want to do, where their passion lies, and what skills they want to develop.

The mentor's effectiveness comes from the protégés trust and respect for the mentor's opinions and judgments. A mentor should always be discrete and never reveal what the protégé confides because difficult situations must be confronted. Mentoring works best when the conversations are confidential from both sides because the mentor needs to be able to share their candid observations. A good mentor, because of a trusting relationship, provides a sense of belonging and reinforces a sense of self worth through affirming the protégé's competence. A mentor is thus serving as a role model, friend, and guide.

Successful mentors should be able, from their personal experience, to suggest how to handle challenging situations the protégé may face with a clear understanding of what is or isn't appropriate given the pharmacy professional norms. A mentor is willing to tell the protégé things they may not want to hear. This self discovery is what empowers the protégé to create the future he or she truly desires. The mentor interacts in ways so that the protégé wants to become better by presenting opportunities and highlighting challenges that might not have been seen otherwise. The supportive mentoring relationship enables the protégé to feel secure enough to take calculated risks because he or she knows what to expect.

Another characteristic of a mentor is someone willing to take the protégé under their wing and share their professional network. This sharing entails introductions and opening professional doors, such as appointments to professional organizational committees, speaking invitations, and other possible mentors. What works best is a two-way committed, enthusiastic relationship in which the mentor gives advice, encouragement, and the space for the protégé to grow and develop, which is attractive to young and current practitioners and thus can serve as recruiting and retention techniques.

Setting Up a Mentoring Program

To establish a departmental mentoring program, clearly identify what outcomes you are trying to achieve. These outcomes might include: reduce hiring time, reduce turnover, or improve satisfaction scores. Be sure you attach specific measurable numbers to the outcomes from data that can easily be tracked on a continuous basis. Reduce hiring time from 2 months to 1 month from the time the position is posted, reduce annual pharmacist turnover from 10 percent to 5 percent, or increase job engagement from 3 to 4 on the 5-point XXY scale used as an organizational employee satisfaction survey are all examples of measurable data. Obviously your outcomes might include having staff trained for the new oncology center, having staff monitoring the development of gene therapy, or using succession planning to ensure vacant leader positions can be filled from internal candidates. You can evolve and change your outcomes as you get experience with the program incorporating new demands. The key is being specific and using measurement. Be sure caring about and helping staff is a consistent part of the departmental culture because if it isn't, regardless of how the program is presented, it will be suspect as self serving for only management.

The next step in setting up a mentoring program is to educate staff and departmental leaders. You want to try and invest in everyone, current and future employees. There are probably many hidden stars already in the staff. Remember that solid performers will appreciate the attention and the ability to demonstrate their capabilities. There are many ways this education might be accomplished. Having a departmental champion who becomes the local expert would be a time-efficient approach. The champion could condense the researched information to that applicable to pharmacy and share. Articles and books such as those listed in the references section is a place to start. Interviews with pharmacy personnel who are or have used mentors will provide useful insights. The staff and managers should talk about what mentoring is —its benefits to pharmacy personnel, what mentors actually do, what makes the mentoring relationship work, and the value to the mentors. Any actual pharmacy stories that may come from hired pharmacy residents, hired new practitioners, or others are very powerful. Having pharmacy speakers who share actual mentoring or protégé experience is one powerful approach.

Once the education is completed, it is time to have discussions between departmental leadership and the staff regarding the mentoring program. Sincerely seek the staffs' input on what is attractive to them about such a program and their ideas about how to structure it. Many issues may come up such as, will it be required or is it voluntary, will participation be included in performance evaluations or salary increase considerations, where will the time come from, why are we doing this? All identified issues should be considered so be sure as many staff as possible have input. Seek out the naysayers and truly listen to them because there may be some pearls in their thinking. Likewise make it safe for the quiet people to share their thinking in one-on-one conversations. If the department has pharmacy interns, residents, or pharmacy students, their questions and input would be invaluable for the recruiting aspect.

Given the knowledge of mentoring and the staff input, the departmental leaders should propose the specific program. The program must be customized and tailored to the desired outcomes and the realities of the workplace. Keeping a list of development opportunities or stretch assignments is helpful. This list could include such opportunities as shadowing senior leaders, organization-wide committees, publication opportunities, speaking opportunities, and program development. Remember mentoring is personal and people want concrete, hands-on feedback from veterans who take a personal interest in them. High achievers have an almost insatiable need to know how they are doing, and the more able they are the keener their need. It is prudent to begin small so it is easy to modify the program given your experience. In the proposal include background, purpose, structure, and evaluation techniques. Try and answer the questions and concerns the staff expressed. Putting the program in writing forces decisions to be made regarding the specifics of it. These decisions can always be changed later but you have to start somewhere. Seeking input from the staff on the specific proposal can fine tune it. Prior to implementing a mentoring program, mentors and protégés must be trained so they can work effectively together.

Training Mentors

Mentors must have a desire to mentor and not just be assigned. Likewise the pairing of mentor and protégé works best when it is voluntary. The success of the mentoring resides in good "personal chemistry" between both parties so there is a comfort level. Letting people get to know each other, not only on a professional but also personal level, can assist in the assessment of the "personal chemistry." Facilitating this knowledge may need to be semi-structured through exercises or workshops. A philosophical approach needs to be shared and role playing with coaching feedback from successful mentors is essential.

Because mentoring involves sharing insights and observations and challenging or encouraging people to think for themselves, examples can be useful. Think of sharing as passing on thoughts, insights, and nuggets of wisdom that creates an atmosphere for good dialog. In sharing, the mentors are letting others learn from what they have learned, both from successes and mistakes. In sharing knowledge and experience, the mentors want to do it strategically with no lecturing, patronizing, or using lines parents might use. Phrases like "here's something you may want to think about or keep in mind," or "have you considered," allows the protégé to try things for themselves. Sharing knowledge and experience through story telling often can encourage the person to share their own stories. The mentor should be sure to share their observations or what they have noticed about the protégé behavior both positive and negative. Frequently affirming what the protégé does right is helpful in these behaviors becoming permanent. These observations spark discussion which invites self-reflection and the opportunity to learn lessons from past performance, such as what to continue to do and what to do better next time. A successful mentor always wants to provide suggestions and resources, not answers.

The mentor is always trying to broaden protégés perspectives. A method to broaden their perspectives is by challenging them to think for themselves. A mentor is often more influential when they ask probing questions versus just providing answers. Asking for plans gives the person the permission and challenge to develop their own ideas, outline their approach, and implement their plan. The mentor's role is thus to provide direction. Asking them for decisions and recommendations stimulates them to evaluate the situation and explore options or consequences of actions. The tools of observation and evaluation assist them in becoming self sufficient. The mentor is moving the protégé along a continuum from where they currently are towards their potential.

Table 1.1 Example. Mentoring Needs Across a Career

Pharmacy Students	Definition of career success (integrated with personal life) Options for practice Obtaining practice experience during School Options for additional education and training (graduate degrees, residencies, fellowships, etc.) How to develop a CV, interview, assess employment opportunities, relocate, enter the workplace, etc. Personal strengths and personal style (working with other styles)
Pharmacy Residents	**Pharmacy Student's Plus** Options for practice or further education or training depending on career goal and personal life desires Professional networks and involvement in professional organizations Teaching and precepting Finding and using other mentors
New Practitioners	**All of the above as appropriate Plus** Revisit and update definition of career success (integrated with personal life) Succeeding in the workplace (culture, superiors, colleagues, other healthcare professionals, etc) Working effectively with superiors Measuring accomplishments and assessing self worth (no longer grades nor closure of semesters/quarters) Being accountable and responsible (leadership) on shift or in practice Life long learning plan Learning from experiences and learning from observing other successful people (good and less desirable)
Mid-career Practitioners	**All of the above as appropriate Plus** Assessment of what currently brings professional satisfaction and challenge Professional dreams that haven't been fulfilled Different things that can supplement current professional satisfaction and challenge The development of action plans with deadlines to achieve any desired changes Being a mentor
Pharmacy Department Leadership Team	**All of the above as appropriate Plus** Depending on job responsibilities, what additional knowledge, skills and abilities are needed to be successful as a leader and how to obtain Switching from pharmacist role to leadership Stresses and how to manage Defining success and accomplishments as a leader What to keep up on now in addition to pharmacy aspects
Veterans	**All of the above as appropriate Plus** Defining what is important now and in the future Desired professional legacy Retirement thinking and needs Part time options, what's attractive

Mentors should not tell protégés what to do, give solutions to problems, make their decisions, give frequent advice, jump in to handle their situations, or criticize mistakes. These actions will kill initiative and self sufficiency, discourage real conversations, and stifle learning to think, although they may be expedient. The mentor's goal is for the protégé to be able to function without the mentor's assistance.

Remember peoples' mentoring needs will change as they progress through their career. Please refer to the Table 1.1 regarding possible needs at each career stage. Frequently ask the protégé for their needs. Evaluate how the mentoring relationship is serving the protégé's needs.

Training Protégés

Some of the mentor training should be adapted to protégé training as is appropriate. Keys to making the mentoring relationship effective involve the protégé taking the responsibility to arrange for on-going time with the mentor. This time doesn't have to be face to face once they get to know each other. Scheduling time together while attending professional meetings can be beneficial if scheduled prior to the meeting to ensure uninterrupted time together. Time away from the workplace will minimize interruptions.

The protégé should also prepare the agenda for time with the mentor so their needs are met. The protégé should think of their mentors as a personal advisory board that they want to keep informed of what is going on in their career and life. They should present their plans and any possible decisions they are contemplating.

Value to Mentor

Paul Pierpaoli in his Mentoring article[1] wrote "Nurturing the growth and self -actualization of a health professional is one of the greatest contributions any of us can make to society."

Mentoring is very much a two-way street, with the mentor also benefiting. A mentor is infected with the enthusiasm of younger people, understands how different generations view things, is stimulated to learn new technology, and realizes how his or her knowledge and experience can help others.

Summary

Given the completive nature of the labor market and the increasing demand for pharmacy personnel, a mentoring program can be a strategic tactic for recruiting and retaining staff. The success of such a program depends on customizing the program to the departmental and organizational needs, training both mentors and protégés, and having specific objectives that can be measured.

References

1. Manasse HR, Speedie MK. Pharmacists, pharmaceuticals, and policy issues shaping the workforce in pharmacy. *Am J Health-Syst Pharm* 2007;64:1292-1293.

2. Pierpaoli PG. Mentors and residency training. *Am J Health-Syst Pharm* 1990;47:112-113.
3. Pierpaoli PG. Mentors and residency training. *Am J Health-Syst Pharm* 1990;47:112-113.
4. Pierpaoli PG. Mentoring. *Am J Health-Syst Pharm* 1992;49:215-217.
5. DeLong TJ, Gabarro JJ, Lees RJ. Why mentoring matters in a hypercompetitive world. *Harvard Bus Rev* 2008;(1):115-121.
6. White SJ, Tryon JE. Success skills for pharmacists: how to find and succeed as a mentor. *Am J Heath-Syst Pharm* 2007;64:1258-1259.
7. Ensher E. Murphy S. Power mentoring: How successful mentors and protégés get the most out of their relationships. San Francisco: Jossey-Bass; 2005.

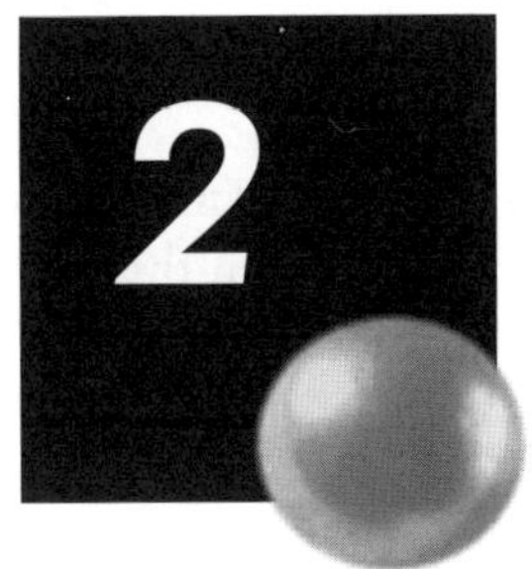

Employing a 360-Degree Performance Tool: Around the Pharmacy in 360 Degrees

Lisa Michener
Stanley S. Kent

Background and Introduction

Continuous feedback is considered invaluable within organizations, especially in managing employee performance. Success in a hospital pharmacy setting is particularly dependent upon continuous feedback between pharmacy management and staff. However, research suggests that the flow of feedback in organizations is typically constrained. Newer employees may tend to be open to feedback in unfamiliar situations or when they fear they are not meeting goals, whereas longer-tenured individuals may solicit less feedback to avoid being perceived as insecure.[1]

The 360-degree feedback method incorporates feedback from all sources with whom the employee interacts, which includes self assessment, reviews from peers, direct reports, managers, and customers.[1] This method is known by many names: multirater or multisource feedback, upward appraisal, coworker feedback, multiperspective ratings, and full-circle ratings. One of the earliest applications of multisource feedback methods dates back to the 1940s when British military intelligence developed an assessment center to determine a candidate's worthiness to act as a foreign intelligence operative.[2] Through history, generational gaps and existing traditional workplace hierarchy limited adoption of 360-degree method in the workplace. However, as organizations shifted focus in the workplace to customer satisfaction, teamwork and empowerment, 360-degree feedback method gained significant momentum. During the 1990s, driven by the advancement of technology for performance assessment, this method became broadly accepted in both public and private industry sectors as an effective and powerful tool to provide a credible assessment of employees and to serve as a means of development and performance improvement for staff.[2]

The 360-degree feedback method has been used in healthcare as a tool to evaluate medical residents' performance[3-8] and also has been validated as a method of evaluating healthcare administrators.[2] An abundance of published work exists in the pharmacy literature that focuses on general methods of conducting performance appraisals.[9-17] This chapter will provide a review of the development, implementation, pitfalls, and successes of the 360-degree feedback method in an inpatient pharmacy environment.

The American Society of Health-System Pharmacists (ASHP) *Guidelines on Recruitment, Selection, and Retention of Pharmacy Personnel* states this method may assist in identifying opportunities for improving management and may also serve to compare management ratings with that of the staff. ASHP further notes that, if not properly managed, the use of this tool can backfire and create animosity among management and employees.[18]

Institution

Glenbrook Hospital is a 143-bed community teaching hospital located in the northern suburbs of Chicago and is one of three hospitals in the Evanston Northwestern Healthcare (ENH) system. ENH is an integrated healthcare system that includes Evanston, Glenbrook, and Highland Park Hospitals, ENH Medical Group (comprising 65 medical offices and facilities), ENH Home Services, ENH Research Institute, and ENH Foundation. The Glenbrook Hospital inpatient pharmacy consists of 30 employees and utilizes an electronic medical record system equipped with computerized physician order entry, bar-coding, unit-based cabinets, and decentralized clinical services.

A 360-degree feedback assessment tool was developed and implemented at Glenbrook Hospital inpatient pharmacy during July 2007. Prior to initiating this new assessment method, ENH used a standard template evaluation for all staff members. The existing evaluation form incorporated elements of the job description, a categorical rating scale for each skill set section and a space for comments. Depending on the job description, this form usually ranged from 5 to 10 pages in length. Using this form, managers evaluated staff, and staff completed self-evaluations. Peer evaluations were also incorporated by some pharmacy managers, but this was not required by the Human Resources (HR) department within ENH. When peer evaluations were used, staff pharmacists completed one evaluation for one other peer in the same job category.

At ENH, performance evaluations are used to determine merit-based pay increases. By corporate policy, annual evaluations for all employees are based on a July-June time period and are conducted during the months of July through September, with subsequent merit increases effective in October. At Glenbrook Hospital inpatient pharmacy, a more efficient tool was desired to assist a new manager in gaining knowledge about the staff's self and peer perceptions that differed from the previously used methods. Two other factors that make management-only evaluation of staff a challenge are decentralized pharmacy services and the fact that the manager's office is physically located away from the pharmacy, thus direct observation of performance is more difficult. At the time of the evaluation, Glenbrook Hospital inpatient pharmacy department consisted of 30 staff members, including one department manager, 12 clinical pharmacists (6 full-time and 6 part-time staff), and 17 technicians (10 full-time and 7 part-time staff).

Before the development of the 360-degree feedback method, the necessity to expand the existing scope of assessment to solicit staff's insight was evident. After in-depth research, the 360-degree feedback method was discovered to be the ideal tool to assist management in understanding staff's perceptions for employee performance, learning the dynamics of the department as a whole, and providing a catalyst for potential staff development opportunities.

Development of the Tool

The main purpose for developing the 360-degree feedback method assessment was to gain insight into staff perceptions of the department that would enhance the existing corporate evaluation process. This process was not intended to replace the existing evaluative assessment or to determine salary adjustments or changes in job status. This approach of using the 360-degree feedback method, for development rather than as the sole performance appraisal, has been advocated in multiple published resources. [19-21]

Although numerous commercially available products are available for this assessment, the pharmacy manager sought to develop a tool internally that would reflect the department's needs. The evaluation form was derived and adapted from multiple assessment forms already in use by the pharmacy department for pharmacist reference confirmation and student and resident assessments. The benefit of using an internally developed instrument is that items selected are deemed most significant to the department locally. Unfortunately, without external validation of reliability, an internally developed instrument lacks normative and validation studies offered by the best commercially available providers. In addition, administration may be more cumbersome with internally developed devices.[19]

After consulting with HR and a pharmacy administrators, it became clear that there were four basic rules to follow:

1. The form needed to be concise—The survey needed to be both concise and easy to understand. A one-page form was essential to keep the staff engaged while completing the assessment. The traditional 5–10 page evaluation used by the department would not provide a well-rounded assessment needed by manager since it represented only one individual's perception of one other employee.
2. The purpose of the evaluation needed to be understood by all staff—The assessment was discussed individually with each employee, informing them why the department was starting the process and answering all questions up front. Staff needed to be at ease with the process to provide candid and sincere communication. It was emphasized to staff members that they were not actually conducting an evaluation of a peer, but rather providing input to the manager so that a better evaluation of performance could be conducted. While this seems to be a fine point of difference, it frames the employee's perception of the process differently and may have human resource implications should an evaluation be challenged.
3. Peer responses would be kept confidential–The decision had to be made early in the process whether completing the form would be required and anonymous for staff. In discussions with HR and pharmacy administration, the decision was made to require all staff to complete the 360-degree feedback method assessment, in addition to the existing required annual self and manager evaluations. In addition, it was decided that all responses would be kept confidential. The identity of the individual would be made known only to the manager. It was believed that a totally anonymous evaluation form would foster the perception of providing comments without ownership or responsibility. The form was not intended to be a lightening rod for all staff's complaints about fellow employees, but rather an honest personal assessment of self, peers, and management. All information was kept in confidence between peers and viewed only by the manager. Furthermore, staff was encouraged to provide critical feedback of all staff members, including the manager, in an attempt to gauge how management was meeting each staff member's needs.
4. The primary goal of the assessment was improvement and development, not to discipline— The assessment's primary goal was for management to "get to know the

Glenbrook Inpatient Pharmacy 360-Degree Method Evaluation

5= Exceeds: Performance exceeds expectations for this responsibility in almost all duties on a sustained basis.
4= Meets Plus: Performance always meets and frequently exceeds expectations in both the quantity and quality of work.
3= Meets: Performance meets expectations for this responsibility in almost all duties and may occasionally exceed expectations.
2= Meets Minus: Performance meets expectations some of the time for this responsibility.
1= Does not Meet: Performance is below expectations for this responsibility. Immediate improvement is necessary.
0= Not Applicable: Rating reserved for those responsibilities and duties that do not specifically apply to this employee.

FILL IN SCORE UNDER PERSON'S NAME	Rph/ Tech1	Rph/ Tech2	Rph/ Tech3	Rph/ Tech4	Rph/ Tech5	Rph/ Tech6	Rph/ Tech7	Rph/ Tech8	Rph/ Tech9	Rph/ Tech10	Rph/ Tech11	Rph/ Tech12	Rph/ Tech13	Rph/ Tech14	Rph/ Tech15	Rph/ Tech16	Rph/ Tech17
Is dependable and trustworthy																	
Willingly accepts assigned tasks																	
Works well to solve problems independently																	
Completes work on time / follows through on work																	
Helped others with their work when needed																	
Does work accurately and completely																	
Works well with others																	
Is a valuable member of the team overall																	
Is easy to communicate with/approachable																	
Add Up & Enter Total Scores Here																	

COMMENTS: If you a score someone LESS THAN 2, Please COMMENT below in the improvement section below or on the back of this page.

	Tell me one thing this person does well.	**Tell me one thing this person can improve upon.**
Rph/Tech1		
Rph/Tech2		
Rph/Tech3		
Rph/Tech4		
Rph/Tech5		
Rph/Tech6		
Rph/Tech7		
Rph/Tech8		
Rph/Tech9		
Rph/Tech10		
Rph/Tech11		
Rph/Tech12		
Rph/Tech13		
Rph/Tech14		
Rph/Tech15		
Rph/Tech16		
Rph/Tech17		

Figure 2.1. 360-Degree method evaluation form.

staff"— a learning tool for improvement and development in the department rather than a punitive measure. Staff was assured that critical feedback would not be taken personally but rather that it would be used to understand what could be done to foster a better departmental environment.

Using the Tool

The evaluation form was divided into a numerical section and a section for narrative comment. All items on the evaluation were reviewed and approved with HR and a pharmacy administrator. After brainstorming on a bank of possible assessment elements, nine items were chosen. The nine items were selected because they were the most succinct and straightforward items for peer assessment

Each employee rated the specific attributes using the categorical scale already in place in the ENH corporate evaluation form. Each item in the categorical scale was assigned numerically on a scale from 1–5, ranging from 1 = does not meet to 5 = exceeds (Fig. 2.1). If the employee did not feel they had enough interaction with the peer to make a meaningful assessment, they could rate the item with a 0 (not applicable). However, if an employee scored their peer with less than 2, they were asked to provide comments in the narrative section.

In the narrative section, each employee was asked to provide a statement of "one thing the individual does well" and "one thing the person could improve upon." The employee was also given the back side of the form to include any additional explanatory comments if desired (Fig. 2.1).

In the first trial of the evaluation, it was decided to have pharmacists rate each other on one form and the technicians rate each other on a separate form. As recommended by HR and pharmacy administrator, the manager also was part of this process and had to complete a self- evaluation in addition to the 360-degree feedback assessment. Each employee was given 2 weeks to complete evaluation forms.

Statistical Analysis

All ratings were collected on paper from each staff member and then entered into a Microsoft Excel ® Spreadsheet. Numerical ratings for the nine questions were averaged for each individual

Table 2.1. Pharmacist Numerical Descriptive Statistics for Mean Evaluation Scores

Evaluation	n	Mean	Std Dev	Minimum	Maximum
Manager	13	4	0.5	2.9	4.9
Peer	13	4.4	0.4	3.2	4.8
Self	13	3.6	0.3	2.9	3.9

Table 2.2. ANOVA Comparing Mean Scores: Pharmacists

Evaluation	Evaluation	Estimate	Standard Error	Adj P
Manager	Peer	-0.3746	0.08233	0.0018
Manager	Self	0.4808	0.1642	0.0316
Peer	Self	0.8554	0.1373	0.0001

who completed the evaluation to form a composite score. Descriptive statistics were generated using SAS® version 9.1. Pharmacist peer ratings were analyzed separately from technician peer ratings. A repeated analysis of variance (ANOVA) comparing means and Tukey's post-hoc adjustment for pair-wise mean comparison was performed. The agreement between raters was evaluated using the means concordance correlation. Means concordance correlation demonstrates whether groups of rater assessments agree. Linear regression was performed between the group ratings to assess the findings from means concordance correlation coefficient. Finally, internal validity of manager scores was assessed using Cronbach's alpha. Cronbach's alpha demonstrates whether the questions being asked are measuring the same phenomena, in this case employee performance.

Results

Pharmacist Evaluation

Overall, mean scores were highest in peer evaluations (mean=4.5), followed by manager (mean=4), and then self (mean=3.6). Standard deviations between scores were similar between the three groups (manager=2.9 to 4.9; peer= 3.2 to 4.8; self= 2.9 to 3.9) (Table 2.1). Mean scores were different among evaluations from manager, peer, and self ($p<0.0001$) (Table 2.2).

Table 2.3. Technician Numerical Descriptive Statistics for Average Score

Evaluation	n	Mean	Std Dev	Minimum	Maximum
Manager	17	3.7	0.7	2.2	4.8
Peer	17	4.5	0.5	3.7	5
Self	17	3.9	0.4	3.2	4.5

In the pharmacist survey, we found a significant agreement between manager and peer evaluation mean scores (concordance correlation coefficient=0.618; 95% CI 0.354, 0.883). Linear regression of manager evaluation and peer evaluation scores revealed a relationship consistent with the concordance correlation coefficient (non-zero slope, p=0.007)). The slope was not significantly different from 1 (p=0.8889), further supporting agreement between the peer and manager evaluations.

Technician Evaluation

In technician evaluations, mean scores were highest in peer evaluations (mean=4.5) followed by self-assessment mean scores (mean=3.9) and then manager scores (mean=3.7). Standard deviations were again similar between the three groups (manager=2.2 to 4.8; peer=3.7 to 5; self=3.2 to 4.5) (Table 2.3). The mean score between manager and self assessments did not differ significantly (Table 2.4).

A moderate agreement was seen between self and peer evaluations for technician surveys (concordance correlation coefficient=0.423; 95% CI 0.205, 0.641). Linear regression of self evaluation and peer evaluation revealed a non-zero slope (p=0.0001) that was not significantly different from 0.9 (p=0.0864), but was found to be somewhat smaller than 1 (p=0.0189). This demonstrates that self and peer evaluations tended to agree with one another.

Internal Validity of 360-Degree Feedback Method

Using manager evaluation scores, in pharmacist evaluations (n=13) the Cronbach's alpha was 0.751; in technician evaluations (n=17), Cronbach's alpha was 0.795. When combining both samples (n=30), the Cronbach's alpha was 0.776. In general, a Cronbach's alpha of 0.7 or greater shows an acceptable level of internal consistency. Therefore, it can be concluded that the nine questions were internally consistent to measure the employees' performance.

Advantages and 360-Degree Feedback Method

An extensive body of literature focuses on the advantages of 360-degree feedback method. Commonly provided examples of benefits include:

Table 2.4. ANOVA Comparing Mean Scores: Technicians

Evaluator	Evaluator	Estimate	Standard Error	Adj P
Manager	Peer	-0.7624	0.1593	0.0006
Manager	Self	-0.2088	0.152	0.3773
Manager	Self	0.5535	0.06459	<.0001

1. Enables management to incorporate staff perceptions into the evaluative process
2. Enhances two-way communication giving the employee opportunity for involvement
3. Shows employees their opinions count
4. Can improve teamwork within the organization
5. Could positively affect managerial performance[24]

The 360-degree feedback method enables management to incorporate staff perceptions into the evaluative process. In addition, new department managers will not always know an individual employee's performance, and if delivered effectively, this method can provide information previously unavailable to the manager. Finally, this process also gives the opportunity to the manager to compare and contrast his or her own views about staff perceptions.

Disadvantages of 360-Degree Feedback Method

Although much of the literature extols the virtue of the 360-degree feedback method, improper execution of this method will not succeed and can foster animosity among staff.[2, 18, 20-22] Examples of mistakes managers make when executing 360-degree feedback method include: lack of a definite purpose, failure to conduct a pilot test and evaluate effectiveness, use of 360-degree feedback method to manage poor performance, inadequate resources available to staff, unclear objectives to staff, and failure to involve key stakeholders.[22] Negative feedback to staff can also be construed as unconstructive when the origin is not made clear. This negative feedback can undermine teamwork that previously existed in the department.

Fortunately, these mistakes were anticipated and avoided in this case. The defined strategy and objective of the new process was made clear up front with staff members: it was to be used it as a learning tool to incorporate into the existing evaluative process and not intended for disciplinary action of poor performance. To ensure that adequate resources were available, each staff member was individually engaged in the process and given the opportunity to ask questions before and after completing the evaluation. This chapter highlights the initial pilot of this process. Furthermore, the key stakeholders who were involved in setting up the initial evaluation included HR and pharmacy administration.[22]

Discussion

In this process scores across the three groups (manager, self, and peer) showed variability that is consistent with published literature.[22] There were no major outliers in the assessments in comparing the manager's feedback to that of peer assessments. This observation was both comforting and affirming to the pharmacy manager. Based on the interpersonal relationships known to the manager, the agreement between manager and peer scores in the pharmacist groups and between peer and self scores in the technician group did not come completely as a surprise. Based on the manager's perception, the lowest performers seemed to provide the least objective numerical and narrative responses. The highest performers in the department provided the most specific, thorough, and detailed responses that were useful to the manager.

Evidence suggests that self-ratings can be often inflated, unreliable, invalid, and biased when compared to the ratings of others.[24-25] Self-ratings can differ from other ratings and do not necessarily relate to employee performance. Because self evaluations may be inflated, *alone* they do not necessarily provide vital information.[20] However, self-evaluations may be used to judge the employee's self-awareness, and this may indicate an employee's future success with an organization.[23]

Limitations

Because this evaluation was not anonymous, the assessments may not have been completely honest or candid.[22] In the initial stages of development, it was believed that the 360-degree feedback method should be completely anonymous. Results of making peer scores available to all staff may tend to increase scores and decrease overall variance and accuracy.[23] In addition, staff may fear retribution, if their identity is revealed. It is possible that individual staff members did not express their true opinions because the manager was made aware of their identity. However, after weighing the risk of this possibility, it was decided that complete anonymity could limit the staff perception of accountability of their feedback, and this was a calculated risk the management took in conducting the assessment.

Given the limited department size, the sample used in the numeric analysis did not provide a robust measurement of statistical reliability, reproducibility, or inter-rater agreement. Finally, using mean scores limits the ability to observe differences between individuals for separate items.

Numerical analysis was in some ways less informative compared to individual narrative comments provided by staff. Staff seemed to provide candid responses in the narrative portion, even when, numerically, the responses were neutral. The narrative description of staff was compared with that of the manager to subjectively assess consistency. Information gained from this process was deemed particularly valuable to the manager in understanding interpersonal opinions in the department and whether the manager had correct perceptions. Finally, new areas for growth potential were observed for individual staff members as well as for the manager. Opportunities for improving teamwork and communication were also revealed.

Next Steps

In this pilot, the numerical results were used in conjunction to the narrative comments to examine staff perceptions. Taken in this integrated context, the results were found to be useful and enlightening to the new manager. Moving forward, with the addition of new staff as well as management, this method will be blended into the existing corporate evaluative process at Glenbrook Hospital inpatient pharmacy. In the future, plans will incorporate technology (online survey development tools) to assist in simplifying survey development and providing metrics analysis and summary

Conclusion

Although feedback provided was subjective, the 360-degree feedback method provided objectivity by allowing the manager to compare employee peer evaluations ratings with that of the manager.

The evaluations were helpful in developing individual action plans for staff development and also enlightening in forming departmental goals for new management staff. In conclusion, the 360-degree feedback method can, in conjunction with other evaluative methods, provide an additional tool to the manager to assist in providing feedback that effectively engages the staff's perceptions into the process.

References

1. Ashford SJ, Feedback seeking in individual adaptation: a resource perspective. *Acad Manage* 1989; 29, 465-487.
2. Edwards MR, Ewen AJ. American *360° Feedback: The Powerful New Model for Employee Assessment & Performance Improvement.* New York, NY: Management Association;1996.
3. Evans R, Elwyn G, Edwards. Review of instruments for peer assessment of physicians. *Br Med J* 1994;328:1-5.
4. Popovich J. Multidimensional performance measurement. *J Nurs Care Qual* 1998;12:14-21.
5. Musick DW, McDowell SM, Clark N, et al. Pilot study of a 360- degree assessment instrument for physical medicine and rehabilitation residency programs. *Am J Phys Med Rehab* 2003;82:394-402.
6. Garman AN, Tyler JL, Darnall JS. Development and validation of a 360-degree-feedback instrument for healthcare administrators. *J Healthcare Manage* 2004;49:307-322.
7. Joshi R, Ling FW, Jaeger J. Assessment of a 360-degree instrument to evaluate residents' competency in interpersonal and communication skills *Acad Med* 2004;79:458–463.
8. Massagli TL, Carline JD. Reliability of a 360-degree evaluation to assess resident competence. *Am J Phys Med Rehab* 2007;86:845–852.
9. Coarse JF, Kubica AJ. Objective-focused approach for appraising the performance of institutional pharmacists. *Am J Health-Syst Pharm* 1979;36: 1676-1682.
10. Swartz AJ. Staff evaluation. *Am J Health-Syst Pharm* 1979;36:187-193.
11. Oleen MA. Evaluating the performance of technician trainees. *Am J Health-Syst Pharm* 1982; 39: 814-817.
12. Milewski R, McKercher PL. Impact of peer performance-evaluation on job satisfaction *Am J Health-Syst Pharm* 1983;40:1202-1205.
13. Ross SR. Developing performance-appraisal systems *Am J Health-Syst Pharm* 1984;41: 1567-1573.
14. Schumock GT, Leister KA, Edwards D, et al. Method for evaluating performance of clinical pharmacists. *Am J Health-Syst Pharm* 1990;47:127-131.
15. Chrymko MM. How to do a performance appraisal. *Am J Health-Syst Pharm* 1991;48: 2600-2601.
16. Rao, V, Rascati, KL. Staff pharmacists' opinions about performance appraisals. *Am J Health-Syst Pharm* 1993;50:1181-1185.
17. Roberts MB, Keith MR. Implementing a performance evaluation system in a correctional managed care pharmacy *Am J Health-Syst Pharm* 2002;59:1097-1104.
18. American Society of Health-System Pharmacists. ASHP guidelines on the recruitment, selection, and retention of pharmacy personnel. *Am J Health-Syst Pharm* 2003; 60:587-93.

19. Grote D. Identifying Individual Development Needs: 360-Degree Feedback. In: *The Complete Guide to Performance Appraisal.* New York, NY: American Management Association, 1996:281-341.
20. Bacal R. Documenting Performance-Narrative Critical Incident, MBO, 360-Degree Feedback, and Other Methods. In: *Manager's Guide to Performance Reviews.* New York, NY: McGraw-Hill, 2004:66-85.
21. Arthur D. Gathering Information: 360-Degree Evaluation. In: *The First-Time Manager's Guide to Performance Appraisals.* New York, NY: American Management Association, 2008:39-47.
22. Wimer S, Nowack KM. 13 common mistakes using 360-degree feedback. T*raining Develop* 1998;52:69-79.
23. Eichinger RW, Lombardo MM. Knowledge summary series: 360-degree assessment. *Hum Res Plan* 2003;24-44.
24. Garavan TN, Morley M, Flynn M. 360 degree feedback: its role in employee development. *J Manage Develop 1997:134-146.*
25. Ashford SJ. Feedback seeking in individual adaptation: a resource perspective. *Acad Manage* 1989:29;465-487.

3 Journal Club Makeover

Michael A. Fotis

A student journal club can be interesting and useful to preceptors and practitioners and of high value to students. Some of the problems with student presentations are: 1) the presentations take too long; 2) students read from the paper; 3) the paper itself is not very interesting; 4) students are overwhelmed by statistics; and 5) students are reluctant to state or have not yet formed their own interpretations.

As a preceptor and drug information manager, the following presentation format helps students to avoid fact restatement and promote critical thinking. The result is a more interesting and educational experience for preceptor and student alike.

Get to the Point

We do not help our students prepare for practice if we teach them to take an hour to summarize an article. As a healthcare provider, you have one sentence, two if you are lucky, to convince your audience that you are worth listening to.

Recommended Presentation Overview

For journal club, answer these questions in **one or two sentences.** Students should always use their own words to establish that they have comprehension of the material.

- Why did you pick *this* article?
- Why should I care? (Some people refer to this as an introduction)
- How did they do it? (Methods)
- What did they find? (Results)
- Why should I believe them? (Internal and External Validity)
- What is YOUR conclusion? (Critical Thinking)
- What are you going to do about it? (Why Bother?)

Do not:

- Read from the article or from your handout

- Read entire tables or figures to the audience
- Include superfluous or irrelevant information in your discussion
- Exceed 20 minutes

Recommended Structure of the Presentation

Introduction

Why did you select this article? There are four criteria to use when selecting an article to review and present.

- Everyone is talking about the article.
- The article skewers a sacred cow (these are so much fun).
- There is personal interest in the topic or authors.
- The article is a cheap trashy daytime TV type (my personal favorite).

Demographics

In the traditional presentation, the student assumes a passive role and often reads the entire demographic table to the audience. This is painful for preceptors and other audience members. In the proposed structure, the student summarizes his interpretation of the demographic information. For example: "as you can see from Table 1, there was a good match between the control and treatment group." The student should use examples to support her assessment.

Inclusion and Exclusion Criteria

In the traditional presentation, once again the student assumes a passive role and usually reads the entire listing of criteria to the audience. In the proposed structure, the student presents her own assessment of the inclusion and exclusion criteria and identifies the potential for introduction of bias. For example:" The exclusion criteria are listed on page xxxx - since this study of heart failure treatments excluded patients over 55, I really do not think we can generalize these results to our practice."

Results

In the traditional presentation, the student usually reads the entire results table to the audience. By this point, many preceptors are dangerously close to the maximum daily dose of acetaminophen. In the proposed structure, the student presents his assessment of the results. The results assessment should include whether the results are clinical outcomes (mortality), intermediate results (patient laboratory values), or even mechanistic findings (MIC data). The assessment should also include whether obvious comparisons are missing. For example, "The authors state that cardiovascular complications were measured but this outcome is NOT reported in the results section." As a rule the student should identify the key findings while superfluous material is omitted.

Statistics and Research Methods

Students who can answer the following questions have acceptable baseline knowledge of statistics and research methods.

- What is the meaning of Power, when is Power critically important, and where in the paper can you find the power statement? (Power is critically important in studies claiming equivalence or no difference.)
- Why is intent to treat important? (Drop outs may have experienced more side effects, or failed to respond to their treatments.)
- Explain 95% Confidence Intervals?
- Explain the importance of Number Needed to Treat? How do you calculate the NNT?
- What is the difference between statistical significance and clinical significance? Can you give an example of each?

What is the difference between a case report, case series, case control study, cohort study, and randomized controlled trial? What are the benefits and limitations for each type of design?[1]

Another helpful exercise for students is to give an example for each of the following:

- Inserting bias in the abstract (A stronger conclusion is found in the abstract than in the text of the paper.)
- Inserting bias during allocation (Inadequate blinding steering healthier subjects to one of the study groups.)
- Inserting bias using inclusion/exclusion criteria (Use of these criteria to steer healthier subjects to the study group.)
- Inserting bias when reporting adverse effects (Failure to report adverse effects at all; reliance on voluntary reporting by subjects; use of an incomplete checklist.)
- Inserting bias when measuring efficacy (Use of lab values, mechanistic values rather than clinical outcomes; use of a scoring system omitting key measurements; redefining efficacy to meet study results.)
- Inserting bias in results (Combining severe and moderate adverse results under a single benign term, such as cardiovascular effects, use of relative benefit rather than NNT.)

Study Conclusion

What is your conclusion? Compare your conclusion to the stated conclusion of the authors. (The author's conclusion is not supported by the author's methods.)

What Are YOU Going to Do About It?

These recommendations are reviewed with all of the Drug Information Students at Northwestern Memorial Hospital, and we have found that:

- Students appreciate a structured approach and want advice as to how to choose an article.
- Selection of articles is improved.
- Students do NOT read from the article or handout.
- We can help students improve their understanding of statistics, study design, and bias.
- Critical thinking is more evident.
- Since students must present their own assessment about demographics, methods, results, and conclusions, it is easier for preceptors to provide feedback.
- Presentations are kept to 20 minutes.

If you are frustrated by the quality of student or staff journal clubs, why not give this technique a try?

Reference

1. Greenhalgh T. How to read a paper: Papers that summarize other papers. *Br Med J* 1997;315:672-675.

4 Solving the Call-in Conundrum: Help! I Need Somebody!

Elizabeth Schmitz

Background and Introduction

Pharmacist staffing is an interminable issue for pharmacy managers. The pediatric hospital setting provides additional obstacles when recruiting pharmacists. The challenge facing these pediatric pharmacy managers is finding adequate staffing levels from a dwindling pool of applicants. The national pharmacist shortage shows no signs of improving in the future.[1] From that limited applicant group, the majority of applicants go to the retail setting. Among those who are interested in hospital practice, it is an even smaller number who are interested in the pediatric setting.

Unscheduled absences only compound the problem of staffing during a pharmacist shortage. Scheduled leave can be addressed ahead of time, and adequate staffing levels can be maintained. Unscheduled absences typically result in decreased services and scrambling to find coverage.[2] In the summer of 2007, the pharmacy department at Children's Mercy Hospital was facing overlapping maternity leaves in addition to multiple vacation requests. Pharmacy staff members were going to be stretched thin to cover the scheduled absences. The pharmacy management team had to devise a contingency plan to address how to maintain operations when an unscheduled absence occurred during this time period.

Description of the Problem

Children's Mercy Hospitals and Clinics is a 260-bed teaching hospital located in the Kansas City, Missouri metro area. The hospital has five decentralized pharmacy satellites, located in the Emergency Room, the Hematology/ Oncology Unit, the Operating Room, the Neonatal Intensive Care Unit, and the Pediatric Intensive Unit. The inpatient pharmacy is also staffed with an intravenous admixture pharmacist, a charge pharmacist, and an order-entry pharmacist. There are also two decentralized pharmacists who staff the general pediatric floors.

The staffing model was designed to maximize clinical services in high acuity areas, decreasing medication errors and adverse drug reactions.[3, 4] An added benefit of this clinical model is the job satisfaction that is felt when pharmacists are able to use their clinical skills.[5] The pharmacy management team must be creative and proactive in their approach to staffing to maintain these clinical services.

Option #1 - Base 14	
TIME	
700	Med 2
800	CC1
900	IP 1
1000	IP 2
1100	IV
1200	Med 3
1300	Med 1
1400	CC 3
1500	CC 2
1600	Med 4
1700	CC 4
1800	Clean-up
1900-0700	K1/K2/K3

Key

Med (medicine)1 = Hem/Onc (hematology/ oncology) = 4H, hem/onc clinic
Med 2 = Med/surg (surgical) lower
Med 3 = Med/surg upper
Med 4 = OR (Operating room) and RR (recovery room)
CC (critical care) 1 = NICU (neonatal intensive care unit)
CC 2 = PICU (pediatric intensive care unit) 12 hr shift
CC 3 = PICU 8 hr shift
CC 4 = ER (emergency room)
IP (inpatient) 1 = IP 12 = Charge pharmacist
IP 2 = IP 12 = Order entry
IV (intravenous) = IV room
K 1 = IP 12 = charge pharmacist
K 2 = IP 12 = Order entry/ code response
K 3 = PICU 12 = PICU overnight

Figure 4.1. Staffing grid for 14 pharmacists.

The pharmacy management team at Children's Mercy is a diverse group. It consists of the Pharmacy Director, the Assistant Director, the Decentralized Services Manager, the Outpatient Pharmacy Manager, the Home Care Pharmacy Supervisor, the Lead Technician, the Pharmacy Educator, and the Business Manager of the department. There are members who are pharmacists, and members who aren't. Some managers focus on operations, while others focus on clinical issues. The varied backgrounds of the members of the pharmacy management team help the group develop innovative solutions when faced with problems.

The pharmacy management team met in autumn, 2005 to brainstorm ways to address the continuous need of staffing the department. A Recruitment and Retention Committee was formed with representatives from the pharmacy staff and a representative from the pharmacy management team. They met each month to look at the state of the schedule and to aid in recruiting efforts. They also met regularly with a representative from the Human Resources (HR) department. The committee found that most recruitment materials were geared toward nursing, and pharmacists rarely attended career fairs with the HR representative. The Recruitment and Retention Committee created pharmacy-specific recruiting materials and took turns attending career fairs with the HR representative.

The committee then focused on retention. A survey was created by the committee and was distributed to the staff in December, 2005. The survey results showed that pharmacy staff members wanted to participate more in problem solving. They also wanted increased communication between the management team and staff members, especially in regard to making the schedule. They believed that the decentralized services that they provided on the floors and the flexibility of 12-hour shifts were the department's greatest strengths. Many staff members expressed a desire to cross-train to other areas so they could help on busy days.

The survey results contained many creative ideas from staff members regarding scheduling. As a result the pharmacy management team decided to form a pharmacist-led Scheduling Committee. A representative from the management team sat on the committee, but the chairperson was a pharmacist staff member. The chairperson was selected by the management team, and the rest of the members were volunteers from the staff. This was a dynamic and invested group who were able to tackle putting together and maintaining the schedule. The Scheduling Committee started by re-writing the department's scheduling policy, based on the feedback from the staff survey. They came up with different options for staffing holidays, vacation, and leave. These options were submitted to the staff via the Microsoft Outlook program. The voting button function was used to allow staff members to choose the option that they preferred. This resulted in a scheduling policy that had the complete support of the pharmacy staff. The one problem that the Scheduling Committee struggled with was the chaos that ensued whenever someone called-in for their shift. They met in the summer of 2007, to take on the task of dissecting the problem of unscheduled absences.

The committee found that the primary response to a call-in was a desperate search for a body to fill the hole in the schedule. The charge pharmacist for the day would start the process by seeing if anyone wanted to stay and work overtime. They would then start calling employees who were off for the day or who were part-time or as-needed (PRN) status. The pharmacists at Children's Mercy work 12-hour shifts, three days of the week. On any given day, this means there are multiple staff members at home. Twelve-hour shifts are associated with increased staff satisfaction, but performance measures show that error rates increase towards the end of the shift.[6] Studies have also shown the importance of rest days in the 12-hour shift model.[7]

Option #2 – Base 13

TIME		
700	Med 2	Med 2&3 in IP
800	CC1	
900	IP 1	
1000	IP 3	
1100	Med 4	Med 3 in IP
1200	Med 2	
1300	Med 1	
1400	CC 3	
1500	CC 2	
1600	CC 4	
1700	All help	Med 2&3 in IP
1800	Clean-up	
1900-0700	K1/K2/K3	

Key

Med 1 = Hem/Onc = 4H, hem/onc clinic
Med 2 = Med/surg lower
Med 3 = Med/surg upper
Med 4 = OR, RR
CC 1 = NICU
CC 2 = PICU 12's
CC 3 = PICU 8's
CC 4 = ER
IP 1 = IP 12 = Charge pharmacist
IP 3 = IP 8 = OE/cart fill
K 1 = IP 12 = charge pharmacist
K 2 = IP 12 = Order entry/ code response
K 3 = PICU 12 = PICU overnight
* Management to help check carts

Figure 4.2. Staffing grid for 13 pharmacists.

Option #3 – Base 12		
TIME		
700	Med 2	Med 2&3 in IP
800	Med 3	
900	CC 1	CC 1 in IP
1000	IP 3	
1100	Med 4	Med 2&3 in IP
1200	Med 2&3	after rounds
1300	Med 1	
1400	CC 3	
1500	CC 2	
1600	CC 4	
1700	All help	
1800	Clean-up	
1900-0700	K1/K2/K3	

Key

Med 1 = Hem/Onc = 4H, hem/onc clinic
Med 2 = Med/surg lower
Med 3 = Med/surg upper
Med 4 = OR, RR
CC 1 = NICU
CC 2 = PICU 12's
CC 3 = PICU 8's
CC 4 = ER
IP 1 = IP 12 = Charge pharmacist
IP 3 = IP 8 = OE/cart fill
K 1 = IP 12 = charge pharmacist
K 2 = IP 12 = Order entry/code response
K 3 = PICU 12 = PICU overnight
* Management to help check carts

Figure 4.3. Staffing grid for 12 pharmacists.

These concerns were also echoed by the pharmacy staff. The survey from the Recruitment and Retention Committee showed that the pharmacy staff was willing to pick up extra shifts, but they believed this should not be a routine solution because it may lead to fatigue and errors.

The Scheduling Committee also found that PRN staffing was not a reliable option either. Most of the PRN pharmacists had jobs at other institutions and could not pick-up shifts when given short notice. It is also difficult to keep PRN staff oriented on current polices and procedures.[8] The committee quickly realized that continued reliance on overtime and PRN staff was not an ideal long-term solution.

When the charge pharmacist could not find a replacement for the absence, he or she would then turn to the clinical staff and the managers. The pharmacy management team knew the value of the clinical services the department had established. They were afraid that if clinical services were pulled for absences, upper administration would question how vital the services were. In most cases, a manager was pulled into the workflow for the day. This was disruptive to the pharmacy management team and led to many delays in administrative projects. Everyone agreed that there had to be a better solution.

Description of the Solution

The Scheduling Committee began by looking at the specific needs of the department. The ideal solution would cover the department's essential dispensing functions, protect clinical services, protect management time, and be a streamlined process that encouraged teamwork. Feedback from staff members made it clear that they wanted to know exactly what to do when a call-in occurred. They wanted the solution to be organized and well communicated so that all staff members were on the same page.

The existing staffing model had created silos in each clinical area, and very few pharmacists were cross-trained. The pharmacy staff communicated that they would like to start cross-training to be able to help cover other areas of the hospital. All of the pharmacists rotated through the night shift occasionally and believed they were familiar with orders for all areas of the hospital. However, this limited exposure was not enough to make them feel confident in routinely staffing other clinical areas. A plan was immediately implemented to cross-train pharmacists. The department was broken down into teams, a medical team, a critical care team, and an inpatient team. The members of each team would have to be able to staff all areas of the team. This made cross-training a manageable task by building on the skill sets that each pharmacist already had.

The Scheduling Committee then looked at the workload during the 12-hour day shift and broke it down hour by hour for each area. They asked staff members to give them feedback about when they were on rounds, when their order entry volume was the largest, and when they typically had breaks in activity. This gave staff members an opportunity to be involved and gave the ultimate solution support from the staff. The committee put all of the areas together and looked to see when each area could handle the entire order-entry queue and process orders for all floors. This would give each pharmacist daily exposure to orders throughout the hospital. They could put problem orders on hold and ask the pharmacist in that specific area to resolve them and then

Option #4 – Base 11		
TIME		
700	Med 2	Med 2&3 in IP
800	Med 3	
900	Med 1	Med 1 in IP
1000	IP 3	
1100	Med 4	Med 2&3 in IP
1200	Med 2&3	after rounds
1300	CC 4	
1400	CC 3	
1500	CC 1	
1600	CC 4	
1700	All help	
1800	Clean-up	
1900-0700	K1/K2/K3	

Key

Med 1 = Hem/Onc = 4H, hem/onc clinic
Med 2 = Med/surg lower
Med 3 = Med/surg upper
Med 4 = OR, RR
CC 1 = NICU/PICU**
CC 3 = PICU 8's
CC 4 = ER
IP 3 = IP 8 = OE/cart fill
K 1 = IP 12 = charge pharmacist
K 2 = IP 12 = Order entry/code response
K 3 = PICU 12 = PICU overnight
* Management to help check carts
**NICU satellite closed while pharmacist rounds- after rounds, pharmacist returns to NICU satellite

Figure 4.4. Staffing grid for 11 pharmacists.

let them know the solution as a learning pearl. This created a staffing grid base from which to start (Fig. 4.1). It also provided consistent coverage throughout the day. This allowed the pharmacists to walk away from their areas for a few hours each day to cross-train with their teammates.

The committee then looked to see which areas could pick up additional tasks throughout the day. For example, when one person calls in, an inpatient pharmacist would be lost for the day. That role would be divided between the two general pediatric pharmacists (Fig. 4.2). The general pediatric pharmacists would attend clinical rounds, but before rounds, they would help check the medication fill in the inpatient pharmacy. After rounds, they would also help the inpatient area at different times. The pharmacists in the satellites would help cover extra order entry. This would allow them to stay in their satellites to provide clinical services. The managers would also come out to help to check the cart fill. Grids were created to allow for up to three absences (Figs. 4.3 and 4.4). Beyond that number, decentralized services would have to be pulled to adequately provide baseline dispensing functions.

Conclusion

Providing adequate pharmacist staffing in the hospital setting is a problem that is not going to go away for pharmacy managers. Getting staff members involved in maintaining schedules can be an innovative solution. Scheduled absences can be creatively handled and prepared for, but unscheduled absences can undo a carefully constructed schedule. Creating a staffing grid that clearly delineates the roles of all members of the staff can help control the chaos associated with call-ins. In addition to getting everyone on the same page, it protects clinical services and management projects while fostering teamwork. It also helps achieve the ultimate goal—providing the best care to patients.

References

1. Pal S. Pharmacist shortage to worsen in 2020. *US Pharm* 2002;27(12):8.
2. Shiftwork Solutions LLC. Managing absenteeism. Available at: http://www.shift-work.com/information/absences.htm. Accessed March 13, 2008.
3. Bond CA, Raehl CL, Franke T. Clinical pharmacy services, hospital pharmacy staffing, and medication errors in United States hospitals. *Pharmacotherapy* 2002;22(2):134-147.
4. Bond CA, Raehl CL. Clinical pharmacy services, pharmacy staffing, and adverse drug reactions in United States Hospitals. *Pharmacotherapy* 2006;26(6):735-747.
5. Cox ER, Fitzpatrick V. Pharmacist's job satisfaction and perceived utilization of skills. *Am J Health-Syst Pharm* 1999;56(17);1733-1737.
6. Mitchell RJ, Williamson AM. Evaluation of an 8 hour versus a 12 hour shift roster on employees at a power station. *Appl Ergon* 2000;31(1):83-93.
7. Tucker P, Smith L, Macdonald I, et al. Distribution of rest days in 12 hour shift systems: impacts on health, wellbeing, and on shift alertness. *Occup Environ Med* 1999;56:206-214.
8. Stratton KM. Pediatric nurse staffing and quality of care in the hospital setting. *J Nurs Care Qual* 2008;23:105-114.

Suggestions for Easing a New Practitioner into Management: Who Me? A Manager?

Kristi K. Killelea

Background and Introduction

When considering succession planning within a pharmacy department, looking solely to staff in the department who have management experience and/or training might make things look pretty grim. The 2004 American Society of Health-System Pharmacists (ASHP) Scholar-in-Residence raised the question, "Will there be a pharmacy leadership crisis?"[1] In 2006, 87% of respondents to the ASHP Pharmacy Staffing Survey reported they believed there is a moderate to severe shortage of pharmacy managers (directors or assistant directors.) This represented a 13% increase from 2004.[2] There are potential leaders and managers within most pharmacy departments. The challenge is that these individuals might not know it. For most students in pharmacy school, becoming pharmacy managers or directors is not the career path on the top of their lists. To those interested in hospital pharmacy, a clinical path may seem more desirable. Based on my experience as a new practitioner and new manager, several ideas should be considered to help a new practitioner discover and explore his or her interest in management and subsequently ease into this new path.

Suggestions for Easing a New Practitioner into Management

One-Month Management Rotation

If your department offers a pharmacy practice residency, require a minimum of 1-month management rotation.

At the completion of pharmacy school, I had no interest in a career as a pharmacy manager. I chose to complete a pharmacy practice residency at a large, multi-hospital organization in the Midwest. During my time as a resident, I had to complete a 1-month, required management rotation. During this month, I spent time with the director of pharmacy and several other clinical and operation pharmacy managers. I attended almost every meeting they did, assisted with and completed several projects related to management topics, and had many topic discussions about things I never learned in school with the managers. Although it was intense, I would not have considered a management path after the residency program without that experience.

Department Involvement

If you are a clinical pharmacist with even the most remote thought about management or are interested in developing clinical programs, get involved in your department through participation in a quality committee, Joint Commission readiness committee, program implementation, or any other task force or committee. This experience allows you to determine if this is an area of interest for you, teaches you the political climate of the organization, and provides an opportunity to demonstrate your abilities to the pharmacy management.

Potential Managers

If you are a current manager and see potential in one of your clinical pharmacists, get them involved in the department. Upon completion of the residency, I accepted a job as a clinical pharmacist at Evanston Hospital, part of Evanston Northwestern Healthcare (ENH), located in the greater Chicago area. Shortly after I started, I became involved with the pharmacy practice residency as a preceptor-in-training. I was able to use the skills gained as a resident and also learned about being on the other side of a residency program as a preceptor. As time progressed, I eventually became one of the primary preceptors of the General Medicine rotation for our residents, sharing the responsibility with another pharmacist.

Pharmacist Career Ladder

Offer a pharmacist career ladder at your institution.

When I had worked at Evanston for about 6 months, I began to look at our pharmacist career ladder (Fig. 5.1). I submitted a request to become a Level II pharmacist, interviewed, and successfully took one step up the career ladder by taking on responsibility for our departmental performance improvement committee.

Smaller Management Positions

Create smaller management positions to avoid scaring away potential pharmacists.

When one of two clinical pharmacy managers left ENH, the decision was made to split the position into two smaller clinical pharmacy leaders. The clinical leader had management responsibilities over several (four or five) pharmacists and several (two or three) nursing units. Staffing development was also part of the clinical leader position. One of the most attractive features of the position was the combined roll of clinical pharmacist (about 60% of the time) and manager (about 40% of the time). Because I was a newer clinical pharmacist who enjoyed this aspect of my career, but also had a growing interest in management, the position made sense. In addition to assuming this clinical pharmacy leader position, I maintained responsibility for the departmental performance improvement committee.

LEVEL 1: Clinical Pharmacist

Job Responsibilities:

1. Patient Monitoring
2. Direct Patient Care
3. Training & Education
4. Physician Interactions
5. Adverse Drug Event Reporting
6. Clinical Skills
7. Nursing Unit Responsibility

LEVEL II: Clinical Specialist Pharmacist – (non-exempt) meets expectations for all duties of clinical pharmacist and has demonstrated leadership and project management skills. Accepts accountability for coordinating a service or program of the department

LEVEL III: Senior Clinical Specialist Pharmacist – (exempt) meets expectations for all duties of clinical pharmacist. Practiced in relevant pharmacy environment for at least 3 years. Accountability for a significant program(s) or service(s) of the department as determined by the pharmacy management team. Successful performance in all aspects of Clinical Specialist role. Demonstrated ability to achieve desired outcomes.

ADVANCEMENT PROCESS:

- Pharmacist must apply in writing to the Director of Pharmacy for consideration
  - Show evidence that they meet requirements for advancement
  - An interview with the Director will be scheduled
- Probation period
  - As with all promotions or job changes, pharmacists will remain on probation at the new level for three months
  - At the end of the probation period, the pharmacist's performance at the new level will be evaluated. If the pharmacist is not performing at a satisfactory level, the promotion to that level will not be approved and the pharmacist will remain at the previous level.
  - Increases in rate of pay for promotion will occur at the successful completion of probation period

Courtesy of the Department of Pharmacy, Evanston Northwestern Healthcare, Evanston, IL, 2008.

Figure 5.1. Evanston Northwestern Healthcare pharmacist career ladder and advancement process.

Increasing Responsibility Over Time

Move smaller positions into larger positions as time and resources allow.

The movement from clinical leader to clinical manager was gradual. I maintained all my clinical leader responsibilities but added several more pharmacists and nursing units as well as a group of pharmacy technicians to my oversight. I added some operational responsibilities for quality and electronic health record functionality and support. One of the most attractive features of the clinical manager position was that I would still be able to maintain clinical pharmacist responsibility (about 40% of the time) with management responsibilities (about 60% of the time.) In addition to doing something I enjoy, staffing as a clinical pharmacist helps me to relate with my staff and identify areas for improvement because I perform the same duties.

Mentoring

Be a mentor.

Through routine meetings with my director and of our assistant vice president, I learn and grow in my management experience. Personnel management is tough, and it is not taught in most pharmacy schools. Because of the mentoring of our departmental leadership, management is still interesting to me. The make-up of my manager role helps me to impact patients on a much broader scale.

Summary

Interest in pharmacy management is often a gradual transition. My career path has put me in a position in which I can make and influence decisions about what pharmacists will do and the approach they will take to do it. Whether you are a director looking out at your own staff or a pharmacist looking internally to see what path you should take, remember there are more potential pharmacy managers out there; they (you) might just not know it yet.

References

1. White SJ. Will there be a pharmacy leadership crisis? An ASHP Foundation Scholar-in-Residence report. *Am J Health-Syst Pharm* 2005; 62:845-55.
2. Scheckelhoff D, Bush C. 2006 ASHP Pharmacy Staffing Survey Results. www.ashp.org/s_ashp/docs/files/PPM_2006StaffSurvey.pdf (accessed 2008 March 27).

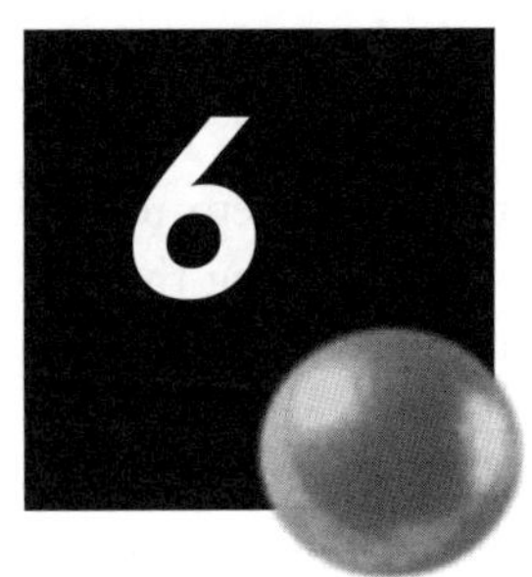

6 Career Renewal: Maintaining Fulfillment and Happiness Throughout a Career

Sara J. White

Introduction

Do you feel at a plateau, stagnant, or stuck in your career? Does your work now seem mundane? Has the work excitement you once had seemed to be gone? Since most pharmacists are in their twenties when they enter practice and will generally work for forty plus years, maintaining fulfillment and happiness throughout a career takes conscious, ongoing effort. Not only does healthcare and pharmacy practice evolve but so does each individual. What made sense when you entered the workplace may no longer be valid, hence the need for career renewal. At some point merely striving to possess things in your life is no longer satisfying and you begin to focus on your internal self, looking for meaning. It is fine to switch gears and move in a different career direction or evolve your current role through this career renewal process.

Career Renewal

Career renewal or reinvention is a periodic reexamination process that can assist you in regaining enthusiasm for your work so you can reach your full potential. In other words, renewal is a way to be the master of one's fate. Think of this reinvention as strategic moves that represent significant and noteworthy movement from your current situation to more desirable work. Make career renewal a conscious choice, a self-initiated goal, and something that you continuously do. In this reexamination process, it is important to reinvent your total lifestyle too because your unhappiness may be coming from conflicts between your career and personal life.

Think of yourself as the CEO, chief executive officer, of your career and life. As CEO you must take charge of being responsible and accountable for your situation. Never feel a victim of your circumstances or blame others, as you always have choices. You are making a choice by doing nothing and suffering in your present situation.

As a corporate CEO you would have others that assist you, such as vice presidents. As a career CEO, every pharmacist should use mentors to help them in managing their career. Seek out other well-respected successful pharmacists and formally ask them to be a mentor. Be sure there is good "personal chemistry" so you are comfortable talking through your candid experiences. A mentor will assist you in clarifying your thinking. Mentors won't provide answers, but through the use of questions help you further your self discovery. It may be appropriate to have several mentors who change over your career. It is critical to maintain frequent contact with your mentor either face to face, via e-mails, phone calls, or internet conferencing. You need to take the initiative to organize the agenda of the time together, share your plans, and discuss anticipated decisions and experiences so you achieve your goals. Likewise you can benefit by merely talking with people who are further along in their career about their experiences and their thinking around the decisions they have or are making. Use professional meetings to meet new people and benefit from their experience. Always exchange business cards so you can contact them later if needed.

The steps in this career renewal process are doing a self assessment, identifying career milestones, and establishing goals-action plans-timelines.

Doing Self Assessment

A self assessment entails setting aside some uninterrupted quiet time to reflect and document where you currently are, such as, your abilities, assets, wants, and desires. In beginning this self-assessment process, it is important to set aside practical concerns, such as family commitments, location, and income so there are no limits imposed on your thinking. These practical aspects can be factored in the process later.

To determine where you currently are, first list your abilities. In other words what do you do well? Perhaps you are good with people, work well on specific projects, or are current in specific disease state therapeutics. Include in this area the kind of person you are. What is your temperament? Are you easy-going, extroverted, or introverted? Do you like to lead or do you prefer following the lead of others? What really brings you satisfaction at this point in your career? What assets of value do you bring to the workplace, such as experience in profile review-order verification, clinical practice, teaching, managing, supervising? Be sure to document your abilities and assets so you can refer to them as needed throughout the renewal process.

To identify your wants and desires make two lists: "*I Want*" list, and "*Twenty Things I Would Love To Do*" list. Examples of items that might be on your "*I Want*" list would be: to feel more engaged at work, to have a lasting impact in my professional life, to retire at age sixty, to teach pharmacy students, to develop a residency training program, to speak at a national meeting, to spend more time with my family. Your "*Twenty Things I Would Love To Do*" list might include: be elected ASHP President, travel internationally, write a book, trace my family genealogy, be a mentor, lecture at a School of Pharmacy, be active in politics. Try and be as clear, specific, and detailed as possible when making these lists. Don't be afraid to dream big and also don't hesitate to include personal aspects as it is impossible to separate a career from a personal life. Nothing is impossible if you put your mind to achieving it. Remember there are no right and wrong answers. Be true to yourself and your desires. Also take into account that your time is not unlimited, and you don't want to have any regrets. Take your reflections and establish career milestones.

Identifying Career Milestones

In setting career milestones be your own career author. Think about your own native energies and desires. Then define your own way of acting on them. Remember when you total up all that you've done and experienced and where you are right now, you have to concede that most of the decisions in your life were yours. Given that you choose where you are, you can choose where you are going and need to consciously do so. If you knew you couldn't fail and there were neither constraints nor obstacles, what would your ideal job consist of?

Another approach to setting career milestones is to establish your definition of career success at this point in your life. Ask yourself, has my definition of success changed since I entered practice or since your last self assessment? What are the things you haven't had the time to do? Where are your unmet needs? To assist your thinking, ask yourself what you want your legacy to be? In other words, what do you want the people you have worked with to remember about you? You create your legacy every day by your actions and relationships versus it coming at the end of a career. Given the legacy you desire, are there changes you need to make to achieve it? Another approach is to identify what you are passionate about, excited about, or care deeply about. A way to identify your passion is to ask if you knew you had a limited time left, how you would spend your time and energy. An additional way to determine your passion is asking in which activities do I lose myself and time flies by almost unnoticed. Your passion may be outside your career and if so ask yourself if there is a way to apply it professionally. Factor all these items into career milestones you establish and document them.

Take your self assessment and factor into your career milestones some things from your "*I Want*" list and "*Twenty Things I Would Love To Do*" list. Another way is to think about where you want your career to be when you are forty, fifty, and sixty. Envision the kind of jobs that will allow you to use your abilities, assets, desires, and wants. Realize that you may need additional training or degrees for these positions. Consider if web-based distance learning can be achieved in your current situation. If the positions don't already exist you may need to negotiate the creation of such a position. Mentors can be helpful in how to approach creating a new position. Be sure to factor in any obligations you have such as family, location, or income. However at some point in your career, these may no longer need to be considered, so evolve your milestones accordingly. Be sure to establish as a milestone your next formal review of your career. Merely documenting milestones isn't quite enough to ensure their achievement.

Developing Goals–Action Plans–Timelines

The final step in career renewal involves developing and documenting goals, action plans, and timelines for the achievement of your career milestones.

Given your ideal jobs, develop specific career goals needed to achieve your milestones. A career goal might be to move into a pharmacy management or leadership position by age 50 or to become a clinical specialist by age 40 or to move to a pharmacy benefit management company by age 60.

Put your goal at the top of a page and list the bite-size action steps you need to complete to achieve your goal. If, for example, your goal is a pharmacy management or leadership position by age 50, some action steps might be as follows:

- Find a leader mentor.
- Determine possible opportunities locally or any openings at my current employer.
- Determine if there are other pharmacists seeking these opportunities.
- Review the current leader position descriptions for the qualifications required and preferred, as well as the responsibilities.
- Determine if you meet the required qualifications or what it will it take to do so.
- Perform a gap analysis of your skills, knowledge, abilities against the position description.
- Ask to participate in a project to see if you really like being a leader.
- Inquire about succession planning and volunteer to be groomed.
- Investigate and complete leadership development opportunities both within or outside the organization, such as continuing education courses, the ASHP Foundation Leadership Academy, etc.
- Research graduate programs, such as MBA, MPH, MS.
- Research training programs, such as Pharmacy Administrative Residencies.
- Set up a reading program in the leadership literature.
- Attend leadership programs, such the ASHP Annual Leadership Conference.

If your goal is to move to a pharmacy benefit management company, your action steps might be as follows:

- Research the pharmacy benefit industry and companies.
- Read annual company reports or drug trends publications from those companies.
- Internet research the industry to find some pharmacists who currently work in the industry and seek them out.
- Find a pharmacy benefit management mentor.
- Interview pharmacy benefit management pharmacists to determine prior experience, hiring qualifications, and employment opportunities.
- Review position descriptions and do a gap analysis.
- Attend PBM workshops or programs or read journals, such as organized by the Academy of Managed Care Pharmacists.
- Work on minimizing your gaps.

Once you are comfortable with your action steps review them for a logical order or prioritization and make any needed adjustments and number them.

The next aspect of this career renewal step is to develop a reasonable timeline for each action step. Be realistic given your other responsibilities and assign a deadline for completion of each step. An exact date will be more effective than merely "one week," because it is specific and clearly indicates when that step needs to be completed. The "one week" depends on when you begin the step and is harder to track and thus it is easier to let the step slide because you are busy. A specific date will indicate whether you are on target, ahead, or behind and thus you can take appropriate action. Don't be too hard on yourself if you miss some deadlines, just either double up your efforts or readjust the deadlines. Never give up because you miss a deadline. You are human, and other things always come along.

Since you have established the goal, and the action plan has deadlines, you want to ensure that you work towards and eventually achieve your goal. One tactic to keep your momentum going is to have the goal, action plan, and deadlines visually in front of you so you see them every day. Weekly assess your progress and plan your "To Do's" for the next week or some reasonable time frame. At the end of the week, review what you achieved and make any appropriate adjustments needed for the following week. Your planning rarely totally goes as planned so just get back on track as soon as possible and adjust the action plan steps and deadlines if needed. Making conscious decisions and having things you want to achieve documented and in front of you is a very powerful technique to keeping you focused. Very few people consistently use this technique, although it will greatly enhance your ability to reach your goals.

Summary

For any pharmacist to be totally satisfied and fulfilled throughout their career, he or she must periodically renew their career. Career renewal involves doing a self assessment, identifying career milestones, and developing goals–action plans–timelines. Be the CEO and author of your career through this ongoing reinvention process.

Suggested Readings

Bridges W. *Creating You and Company.* Reading, MA: Addison-Wesley Longman,1997.

Davidson J. *Reinventing Yourself.* Indianapolis, IN: Alpha Books; 2001.

Gardner JW. *Self-Renewal; The Individual and the Innovative Society.* New York, NY: W.W. Norton Company; 1981.

Mackowiak J, Eckel FM. Career management: an active process. *Am J Health-Syst Pharm* 1985;42:554-560.

White SJ. Success skills for pharmacists: career renewal. *Am J Health-Syst Pharm* 2008;65:119-121.

White SJ. Success skills for pharmacists: Integrating your personal life and career. *Am J Health-Syst Pharm* 2007;64:358-359.

White SJ, Tryon JE. Success skills for pharmacists: how to find and succeed as a mentor. *Am J Health-Syst Pharm* 2007;64:1258-1259.

Part

2

Program Development, Implementation, and Management

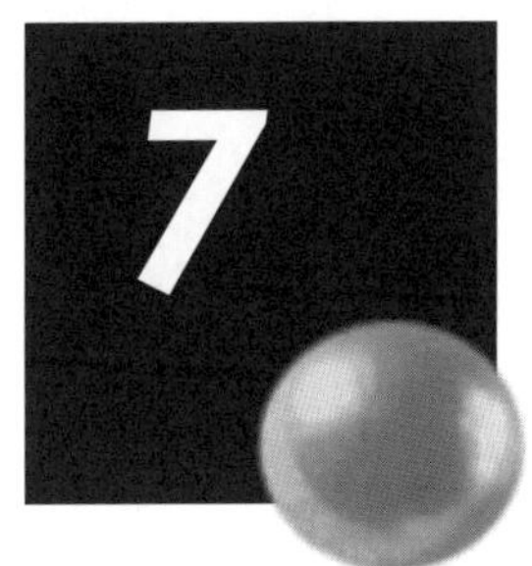

7 Establishing County-Wide Concentration and Dosing Unit Standards for High-Risk IV Medications

John H. Eastham

Introduction and Institution

The San Diego Patient Safety Consortium (SDPSC) consists of participating representatives from hospitals in San Diego County. The group evaluates areas for local inpatient safety improvements. In 2006, the Consortium created a task force to standardize IV medication concentrations and dosage units (i.e., mg/min, mg/kg/min, etc.) in adult San Diego County hospitals.

To create the task force, multi-hospital healthcare systems and stand-alone hospitals were encouraged to provide no more than two participants. Task force participants were pharmacists and nurses who oversaw medication safety and quality. Of 22 adult hospitals in San Diego County, 17 were represented on the task force.

Case for Standardization

The case for IV standardization can be made for several reasons. From a regulatory perspective, the Joint Commission requires minimizing and standardizing injectable medication concentrations within a hospital. The medication safety literature indicates that standardization should be employed whenever appropriate and that IV medications have the highest potential for patient harm. Physicians and temporary/per diem staff may rely on IV dosing units or IV concentrations standards from other institutions because they are more familiar with those standards. Task force members shared their experiences with medication errors occurring in their facilities due to lack of standardization. These examples included a four-fold insulin concentration error, a 60-fold labetalol dosing-unit error, and errors involving smart IV pumps with different drug libraries that were transferred between hospitals of the same system.

Process

Task force members reviewed individual hospital IV concentration and dosing unit standards; in some cases, none had been formalized. References were checked as needed. These refer-

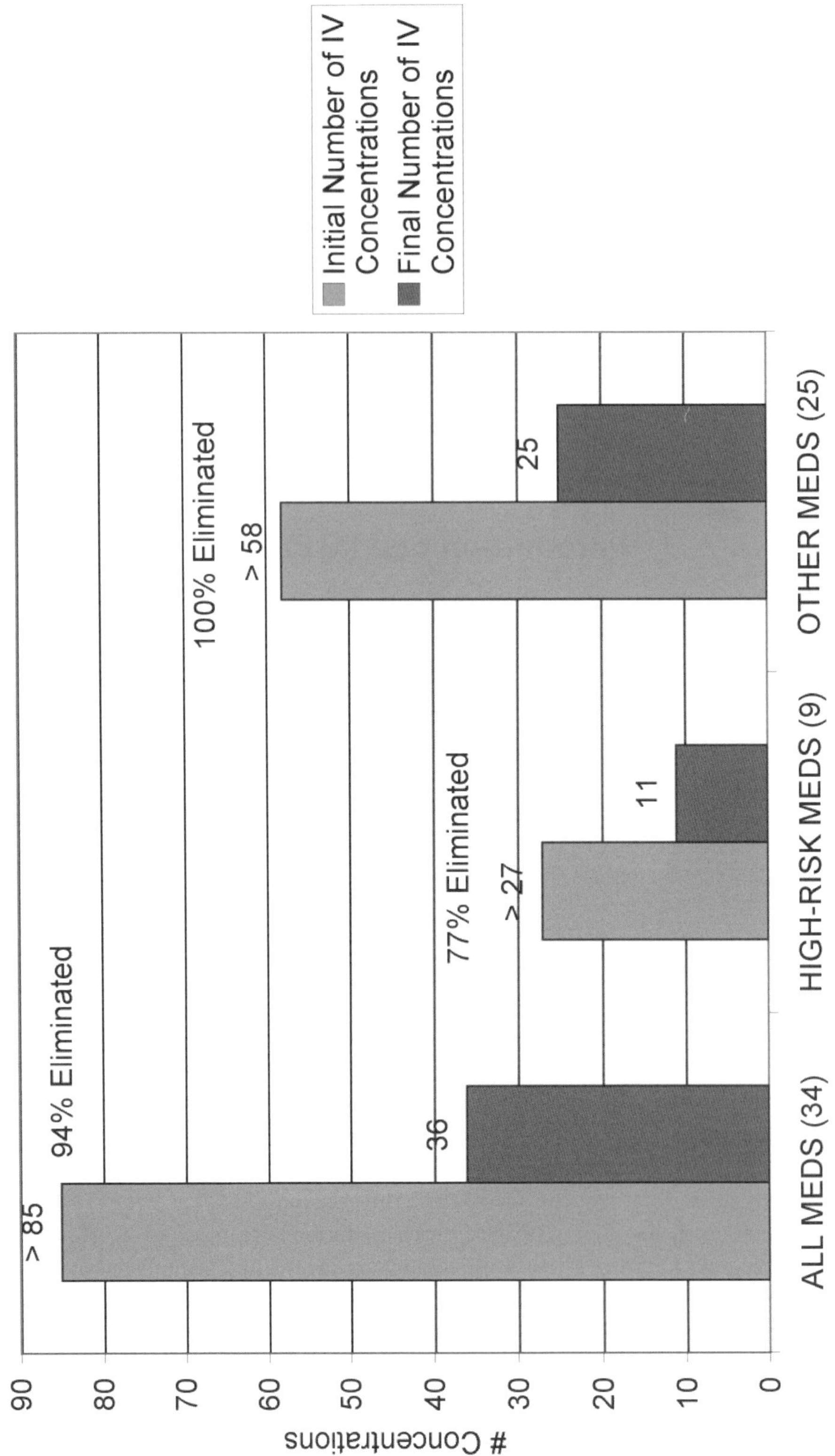

Figure 7.1. Consensus on IV concentration standards.

ences included well-known medication dosing references, manufacturers' recommendations, Society of Critical Care Medicine, and ACLS treatment guidelines. Task force members used a Delphi decision-making process to determine the final drug concentration and dosing unit for each drug. Almost without exception, there was broad consensus for the decisions being made. Champions were also selected from each hospital or system. These champions were committed to make the necessary changes at their facilities. The task force met every other month for approximately seven meetings.

Results

A review of the baseline standards showed remarkable variation between participating hospitals. Some hospitals did not have any formal standard for some IV medications. Overall, of 34 IV medications that were assessed, participating hospitals had over 85 different standard concentrations. Magnesium sulfate (small volume) had six different concentration standards. Magnesium sulfate (large volume), amiodarone, fentanyl, furosemide, and lorazepam each had four different concentration standards.

There was a similar variation in dosage units. The 34 medications reviewed had over 57 different dosing units being used within the participating hospitals. There were four different dosage unit variations for fentanyl, and three different dosage units for dobutamine, epinephrine, and multiple other medications.

After reviewing the 34 IV medications, the task force was able to develop a county-wide standard of 36 concentrations. Because there were more than 85 different concentrations at baseline, there was a 94% elimination in variation for all forms, with 100% elimination for continuous infusions. Nine of these IV medications were considered "high-risk" and included opioids, neuromuscular junction blockers, anticoagulants/antiplatelets, magnesium, and insulin. Concentrations for "high-risk" medications were reduced from more than 27 to 11, a 77% elimination of variation for all forms, with 100% elimination for continuous infusions.

Overall, dosing unit variations were reduced from more than 57 to 34, a 100% elimination of variation. For the nine "high-risk" medications, there were more than 18 different dosing units being used at baseline. This was reduced to nine dosing units.

Adoption Of the Standards

Champions from the participating hospitals and healthcare systems were tasked with making the necessary changes within their facilities. Of the 17 hospitals represented on the task force, 15 were assessed for their adoption of the standards. Of these 15 hospitals, adoption of the concentration standards ranged from 72.2% to 100%. Adoption of the dosing units varied from 84.8% to 100%. Two hospital systems adopted more weight-based dosing units than were included in the standards.

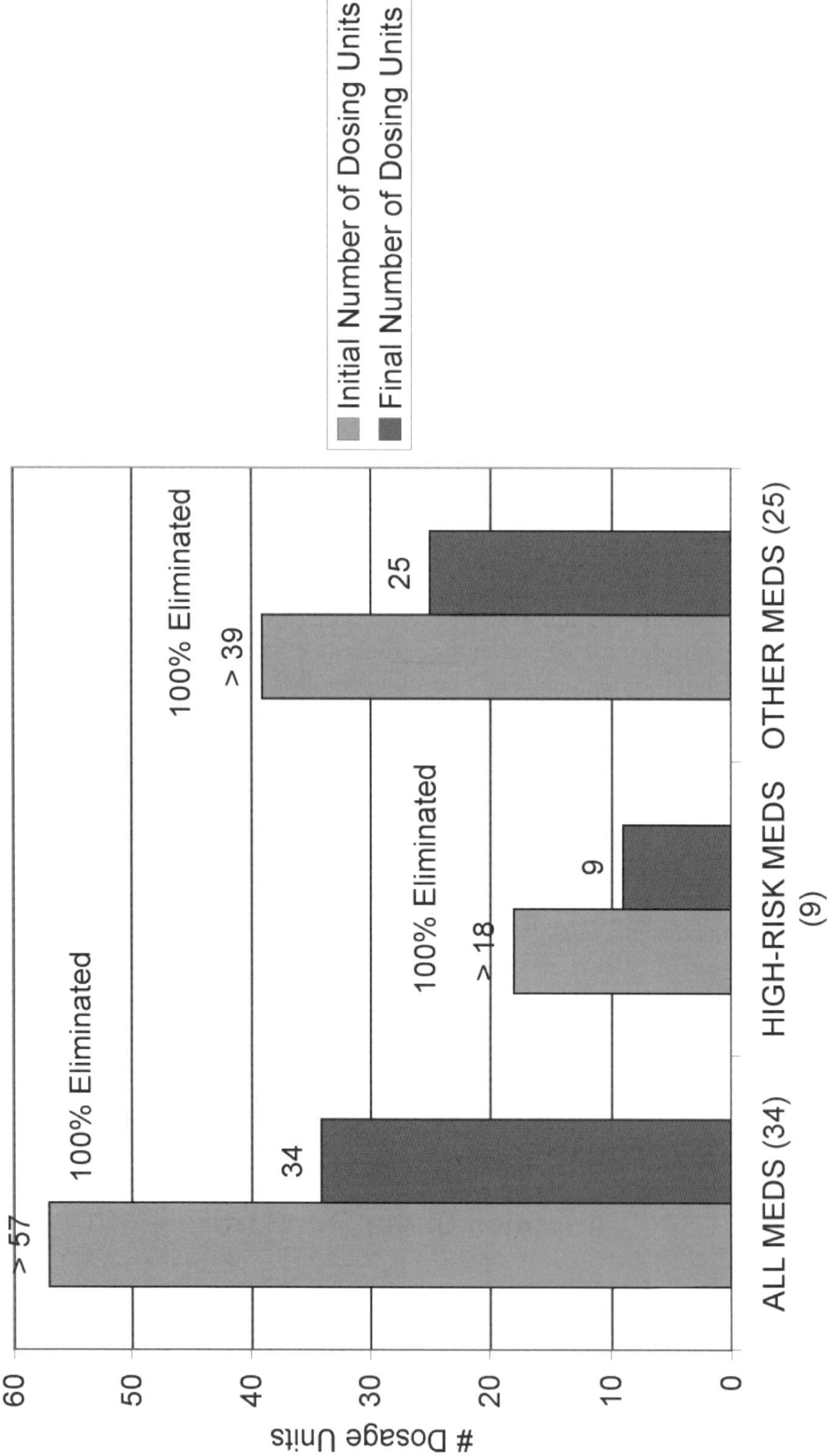

Figure 7.2. Consensus on IV dosing units.

Benefits of a County-Wide Standard

Availability of a county-wide IV standard gave multi-hospital systems the leverage to adopt a single IV standard within their own system. Because smart pump libraries were updated with the same drug library, the risk of medication error from smart pumps with different drug libraries was eliminated.

Following development of the county-wide standards, SDPSC and participating hospitals were the focus of several articles in national healthcare publications, including Inside the Joint Commission, Drug Topics, and the front page of a local newspaper. Although press coverage does not improve patient safety, the articles provided validation of the consortium's efforts, drew leadership's attention to medication safety within participating hospitals, and put indirect pressure on non-participating hospitals to be represented in future SDPSC task forces.

Because most of the task force participants were pharmacists and nurses who oversaw medication safety and quality, the meetings provided an opportunity for networking. The medication safety pharmacists who participated on the task force have developed a high level of professional camaraderie and are actively sharing ideas, strategies, and procedures to assist their peers at other institutions.

Success of the *Safe Administration of High-Risk IV Medications Task Force* has created momentum for future projects, and instead of disbanding, the SDPSC has grown into a new task force focusing on PCA safety, standardization, and improvement.

Findings

After several hospitals adopted the IV standards, champions reported how the adoption process went at their respective institutions. In general, champions began to inform stakeholders within their institutions about the county standards up to a year before the standards were finalized. Extensive education to pharmacy and nursing staff was necessary before concentration changes were made. This education needed to be started about 1 month before any concentration standards were changed. Implementation of the IV concentration (and dosing units, in most cases) standards went smoothly at all hospitals. Since implementation of the standards usually accompanied other changes in the IV management process, it was difficult for the champions to assess the medication error reduction that resulted from adoption of the County standard. A formal risk reduction assessment has not been done. This standardization has been held up by leadership as a model for further standardizations within participating institutions. Two hospital systems adopted more weight-based dosing units than were included in the standards. Reassessing the dosing unit standards and possibly switching to weight-based units has been discussed.

Toolkit Development

Following development of the IV standards, it became clear that other municipalities may want to develop their own IV medication standards. The task force met again to evaluate its experience. Through the support of Cardinal Health, the task force was able to publish the toolkit *Safe Administration of High-Risk IV Medications. Intra- and Inter-Hospital Standardization: Drug Concentrations and Dosage Units. How-to Guide.* The toolkit was designed to be simple and practical. The toolkit can be downloaded at www.cardinal.com/clinicalcenter/materials/taskforce/IVtoolkit.pdf.

Conclusion

Representatives from multiple hospitals and healthcare systems met together to standardize IV concentrations and dosing units throughout San Diego County. There was broad consensus for the decisions being made. Adoption of the IV concentrations standards was high. Adoption of the dosing standards progressed slower, but participating hospitals are committed to adopting these standards. Implementation of the standards usually accompanied other IV management process changes so it was difficult to assess risk reduction.

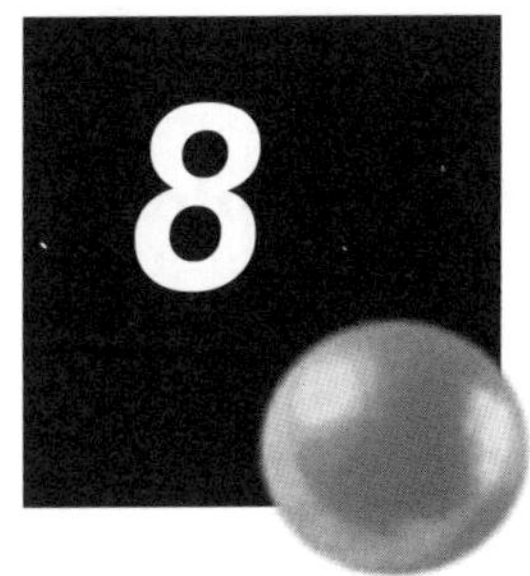

Successes and Challenges of VTE Protocol Implementation

Della Abboud

Background and Introduction

Deep vein thrombosis (DVT) is a condition in which a blood clot forms inside a deep vein, usually located in the calf or thigh. It occurs when the blood clot either partially or completely blocks the flow of blood in the vein. DVT occurs in approximately two million Americans each year.[1] As many as 600,000 people are hospitalized each year for DVT.[2] Symptoms of DVT include pain, tenderness, swelling or discoloration of the affected area, and skin that is warm to the touch. As many as half of all cases of DVT produce minimal symptoms or are completely "silent."

A major complication of DVT is the development of a pulmonary embolism (PE). This condition occurs when the blood clot from the lower extremity breaks loose from the wall of the vein and travels to the lungs, blocking the pulmonary artery or one of its branches. Patients with PE may show signs of shortness of breath, chest pain, rapid pulse, sweating, or bloody cough. Of those patients who develop PE, approximately 300,000 will die each year, more Americans than die from AIDS and breast cancer combined.[3–5]

Deep vein thrombosis and PE both belong to a condition called venous thromboembolism (VTE). Taken together, they constitute an approximately 12% in-hospital case fatality rate[6] and have long been determined to be the number one *preventable* cause of death in hospitalized individuals.[3] More than 200,000 new cases of VTE occur on an annual basis.[7] Thirty percent of these patients will die within the first 30 days.[7] With death occurring in 6% of DVT cases and 12% of PE cases within 1 month of diagnosis,[8] these statistics alone are a compelling reason to focus resources and energy on development of a VTE prophylaxis program.

Hospital

Barnes-Jewish West County Hospital (BJWCH) is a 113-bed acute care facility located in a western suburb of St. Louis, Missouri. The facility offers a variety of specialized services in the fields of bariatric surgery, cardiology, cosmetic surgery, gastroenterology, general surgery, internal medicine, ophthalmology, orthopedics and sports medicine, pain management, physical therapy and rehabilitation, radiology and diagnostic imaging, skilled nursing, sleep disorders, and urology. BJWCH is a member of BJC Healthcare, which is comprised of 13 healthcare facilities in and around the metropolitan St. Louis area.

Venous Thromboembolic Prophylaxis Protocol Implementation

To effectively prepare a plan that encompassed best practices, executive leadership from BJC Healthcare decided to form a system-wide team with representation from as many BJC facilities as possible to share ideas and determine the most appropriate methods for designing and implementing a VTE prophylaxis program. The team included representatives with a diverse knowledge base in nursing, pharmacy, and risk management. The original goal of the team was to develop one process that every facility could implement with success. It did not take long to determine that this goal was not attainable. Although there was strong consensus among the group about the importance of implementing a VTE program, consensus could not be achieved in several areas, including drug selection and scoring methodology on assessment. The group decided that it was not as important to have consistency throughout the BJC Healthcare system as it was to develop a general template that each facility could customize depending on its patient population, physician preferences, and formulary options.

In March of 2006, the first meeting of the BJC VTE System team was held. Representatives from 10 of the system hospitals participated on the team. The first charge of the team was to conduct a literature search to determine how much information was available from outside sources. The goal was to clearly define the various steps of the process, such as design and surveillance of short-term and long-term studies, interventions and their effectiveness, and development and dissemination of education and marketing plans across business units. The team also collected current practices from each of the facilities, including Risk Assessment Forms and Order Forms (Table 8.1).

In May/June 2006, the team was split into four subgroups, each focusing on a different area, as shown in Figure 8.1. The tasks of each group were as follows: 1) Patient Assessment: evaluation of patient risk factors, 2) Patient Assessment: assessment/reassessment across the continuum of care, 3) Intervention and Implementation: physician education, and 4) Intervention and Implementation: patient education. By the end of June 2006, the subgroups had completed their assignments, and the entire team reconvened to share recommendations. The process template was then fine-tuned and rolled out to the participating hospitals.

The process flow diagram in Figure 8.2 shows the steps necessary to ensure appropriate assessment and treatment of all patients upon admission. Once the patient is admitted, the VTE Risk Assessment may be completed one of two ways, either as a nurse-driven process or a physician-driven process. Following the flow diagram to the left outlines the nursing-driven process. The nurse completes the assessment form and determines the patient's risk score. The risk score is communicated with the physician for consideration of the appropriate method of prophylaxis. The physician then reviews the nursing assessment and writes the order for prophylaxis based on the patient risk score. Following the flow diagram to the right outlines the physician-driven process. The physician assesses the patient for the risk of developing VTE either by assigning a risk score or by simply reviewing the risk factors as they relate to the patient. The physician then writes the appropriate form of prophylaxis based on the assessment of the patient's risk. The main difference between the two methods is that in the nurse-driven process, the risk assessment always uses assigned numbers for each risk factor. The nurse calculates the total risk of the patient by adding up the values of the various risk factors to determine the risk stratification for that patient. In the physician-driven process, the scores for each risk factor may be excluded and the physician is able to use more clinical judgment when determining the

Table 8.1. Gantz Chart for DVT Project Timeline

VTE Measurement & Intervention	Feb	March	April	May	June	July	Aug	Sept	Oct	Nov	Dec
Convene team											
Perform literature search & synthesis											
Develop definitions including inclusion and exclusion criteria											
Design method of study/ measurement such as periodic survey (point prevalence), sample (cohort), ongoing											
Implement data management plan for this indicator											
Collect data/ perform study											
Review intervention options											
Analysis											
Intervention development & education plan											
Intervention											
Test intervention effectiveness											

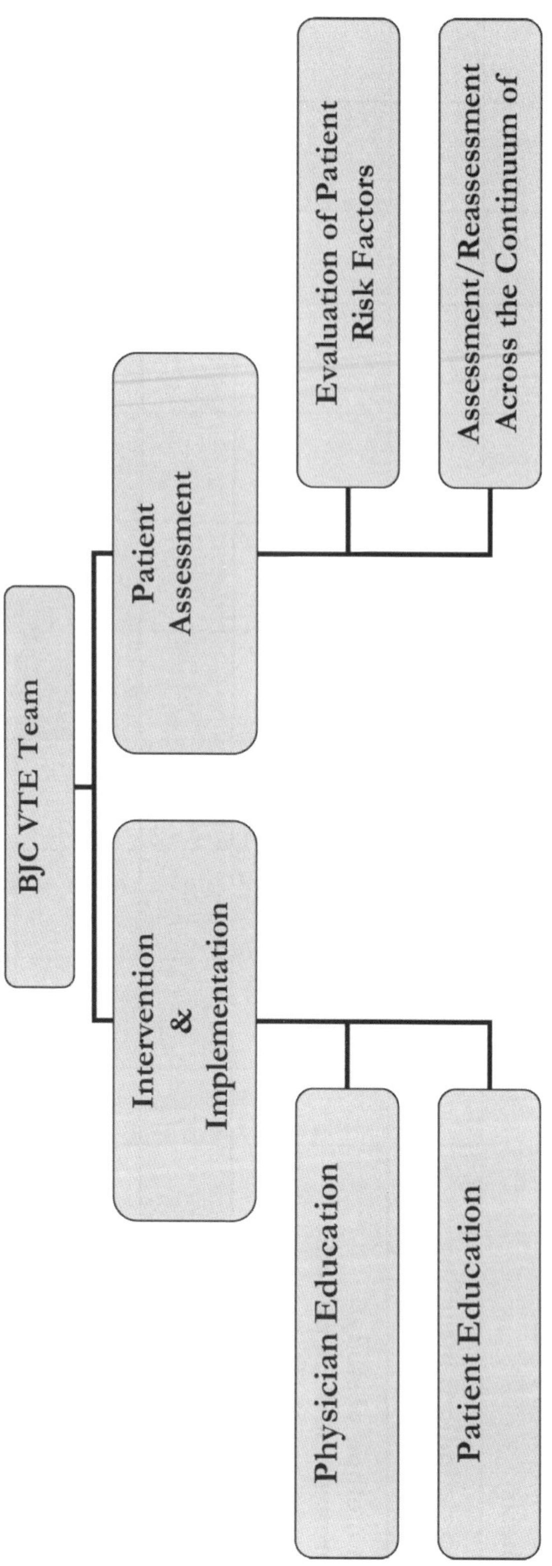

Figure 8.1. Team subgroup development.

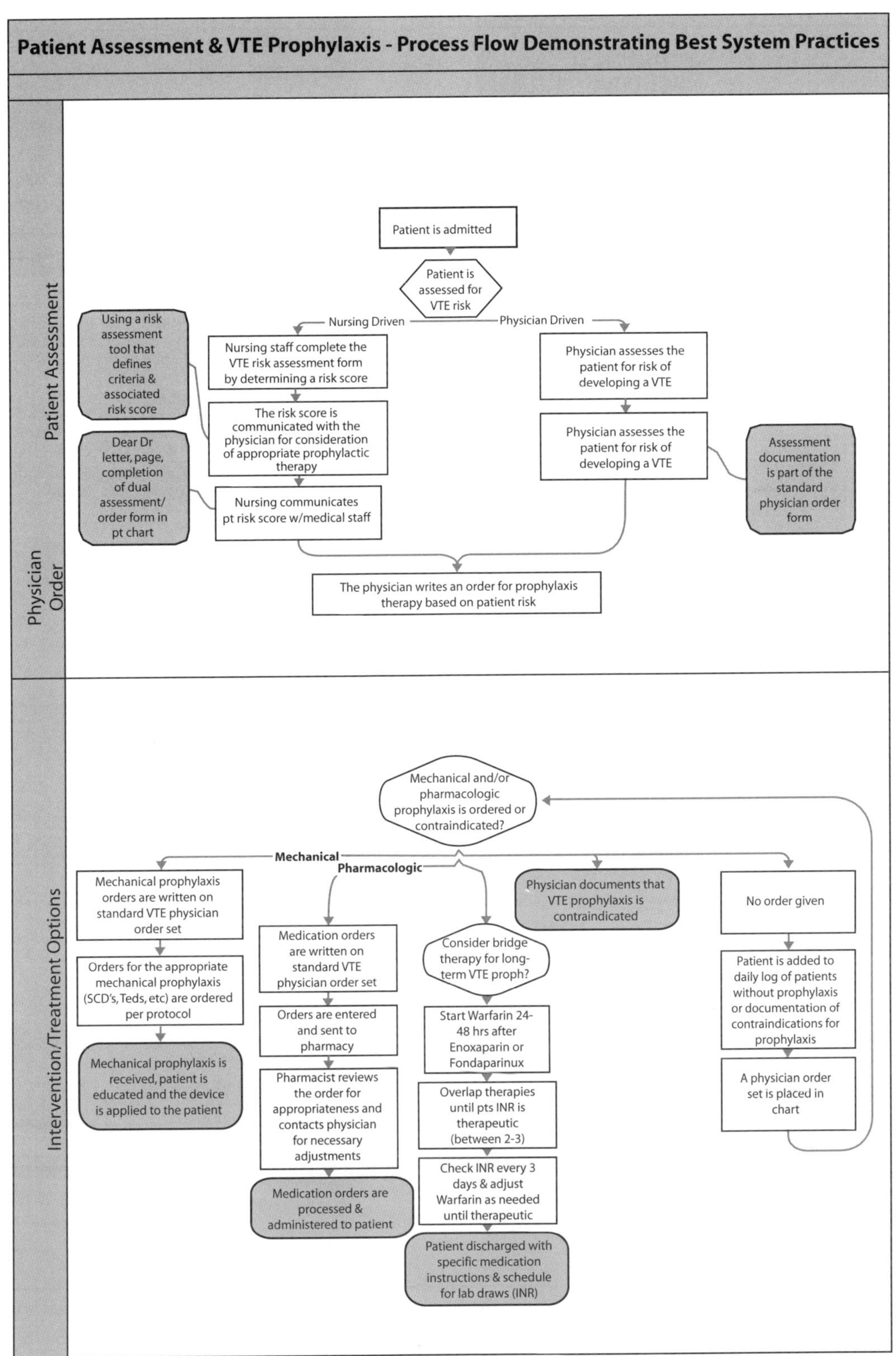

Figure 8.2. Best practice flow diagram for DVT prophylaxis.

Barnes-Jewish
West County Hospital
BJC HealthCare™

INPATIENT DVT PROPHYLAXIS ASSESSMENT/ORDER

ORDERS ON THIS FORM SUPERSEDE ANY ORDERS ON PREPRINTED ORDER FORMS OR WRITTEN PHYSICIAN ORDERS.

ADDRESSOGRAPH

Ambulating (walking in hallways TID) nonoperative patients do not routinely require DVT prophylaxis

Risk factors for immobile & operative patients:
Birth control pills or estrogen replacement therapy
Currently pregnant or postpartum within 6 weeks
Age greater than 40 years
BMI greater than 25 (wt Kg/height cm/height cm x 10,000)
Previous DVT/PE
Family history of DVT/PE
Thrombophilia (congenital or acquired)
Cardiac dysfunction (heart failure, arrhythmia, MI)
Chronic lung disease
Malignancy
Inflammatory disorder (i.e. IBD, lupus)
Swollen legs or varicose veins
Active collagen-vascular disorder
Embolic stroke
Dehydration
Acute respiratory failure
Serious infection
ICU admission or burn greater than 20% BSA
Indwelling central venous catheter
Surgery
Poly trauma or acute spinal cord injury (with deficit)
Spine, hip, pelvic or lower extremity surgery or fracture
CHI (GCS less than 13 not attributable to ETOH or drugs)

Possible exclusion criteria for pharmacologic prophylaxis:

1. Heparin or Enoxaparin Induced Thrombocytopenia (may consider using fondaparinux)
2. Active bleeding (i.e. ICH, active GI bleeding, traumatic)
3. Preoperative within 12 hours or postoperative within 4-8 hours
4. Renal insufficiency (creatinine clearance less than 10 ml/min)
5. Spinal tap or epidural within 6-10 hours
6. Recent intraocular or intracranial surgery
7. Coagulopathy

Physicians are advised to consider other risk factors and conditions for patients that may be contraindications to DVT prophylaxis.

1. Enoxaparin, unfractionated heparin (UFH), fondaparinux, and warfarin are appropriate pharmacologic strategies for DVT prophylaxis.
2. Sequential Compression Device, Plantar Pneumatic Compression, and Graduated Compression Stockings are appropriate mechanical strategies for DVT prophylaxis. An IVC filter may be considered in the highest risk patients with contraindications to anticoagulation.

For Example

Risk Factors	Prophylaxis	If Contraindication exists
0	Early ambulation	SCD
≥1 medical	Enoxaparin 40mg Daily	SCD
≥1 surgical	Enoxaparin 40mg Daily & SCD	SCD

ORDER AREA

I. No Risk Factors Identified

☐ No mechanical or drug prophylaxis required ☐ Ambulate in hallway at least TID ☐ Up in chair and ambulate

II. Risk Factors Identified *(choose one treatment from 1) and one treatment from 2). Consider adding therapy from 3) for patients requiring anticoagulation post-discharge.)*

1) Choose one: ☐ Drug prophylaxis contraindicated due to: ☐ Pt currently receiving treatment for DVT/PE ☐ Pt currently anti-coagulated ☐ thrombocytopenia Other:____________

☐ Enoxaparin 40mg subcut Daily (preferred for medical and general surgical patients)
☐ Enoxaparin 30mg subcut twice daily (preferred for total knee replacement patients)

☐ Heparin 5000 units subcut Q8 hours

☐ Fondaparinux (Arixtra) 2.5mg subcut daily

2) Choose one: ☐ Mechanical prophylaxis contraindicated due to ☐ trauma ☐ vascular insufficiency Other:______
☐ Sequential Compression Device (SCD)
☐ Plantar Pneumatic Compression (PPC)

3.) Optional Bridge Therapy: Warfarin ______ mg 1st dose PO at bedtime today (new orders should be written daily until INR stable and therapeutic).
Patients may be continued on Enoxaparin or Fondaparinux on an outpatient basis without warfarin if determined appropriate by the physician.

III. ☐ **Graduated Compression Stockings (GCS)** (use if risk factors identified but pharmaceutical therapy is contraindicated)

IV. ☐ **Other:**

MD: ________________ ________________ Date/Time: ____________
SIGNATURE REQUIRED PRINTED NAME REQUIRED

DO NOT WRITE BELOW THIS LINE

BWC 6-206 MR (07/19/06) Page 1 of 1

BWC 6-206 MR

Figure 8.3. DVT prophylaxis assessment and order form.

patient's risk stratification. Either way, it is ultimately the physician's responsibility to review the patient risk assessment, determine which method of prophylaxis is appropriate, and write the corresponding order for that treatment.

BJWCH chose to proceed with the physician-driven process. The physician would determine the patient's risk factors but would not assign scores to each factor. The physician would use the assessment portion (upper portion) of the Inpatient DVT Prophylaxis Assessment/Order Form as shown in Figure 8.3 to review the risk factors for each patient.

Looking at the Intervention/Treatment Options section of Figure 8.2 shows the next step in the process flow—determining the appropriate type of prophylaxis, both mechanical and pharmacologic. The physician may also document individual patient contraindications directly on the Order Form. The physician must either order some type of mechanical and pharmacologic prophylaxis or document the reason why no prophylaxis has been ordered. If the VTE Order Form is not completed, the patient's name prints on a daily log, and the physician is contacted to complete the order or provide a contraindication. There must be documentation one way or the other in the chart relating to the use of VTE prophylaxis. This process flow also allows the physician to determine if long-term VTE prophylaxis is needed and suggests overlapping injectable anticoagulants, such as enoxaparin or fondaparinux with warfarin, until appropriate INR levels are achieved, and the patient is ready for discharge.

The order section of the Inpatient DVT Prophylaxis Assessment/Order Form was designed to be as simple for the physicians as possible. It clearly lists all options available to the physician as determined by the BJWCH Pharmacy and Therapeutics Committee. All the physician needs to do is check the appropriate boxes. It is straightforward and takes little time to complete.

Results

Approximately 1 year after implementation, data for all 10 facilities that participated in the original team were collected to determine the impact of the program. Every hospital showed impressive improvement over the baseline data collected prior to implementation of this new process. Many of the facilities had programs in place but were able to improve their existing programs, their compliance, and their rates of appropriate VTE prophylaxis. At BJWCH, we saw a dramatic improvement in appropriate VTE prophylaxis being ordered. The rates climbed from approximately 35% prior to program implementation to approximately 95% after implementation. Through our education efforts, including Physician Bulletins (Fig. 8.4), Grand Rounds presentations, and one-on-one discussions, we obtained buy-in from the majority of the medical staff and executive leadership.

Although we were able to achieve success, future challenges will continue to present themselves. The most immediate challenge includes National Patient Safety Goal 3E, which focuses on the ordering and monitoring of anticoagulants used for treatment. Although the goal states that the focus is treatment doses, it will be difficult to implement a program that involves pharmacists and focuses solely on treatment—essentially ignoring the potential benefits of pharmacist involvement in the prophylaxis realm. Finding the resources to implement and expand these types of pharmacy services will bring us one step closer to achieving our goal of patient-centered or relationship-based care.

DVT: The Road to Prevention

Deep vein thrombosis (DVT) is a condition in which a blood clot forms inside a deep vein, usually located in the calf or thigh. It occurs when the blood clot either partially blocks or completely blocks the flow of blood in the vein. DVT occurs in approximately 2 million Americans per year. This is more than the number of people affected by heart attack and stroke combined. As many as 600,000 people are hospitalized each year for DVT. Only approximately one-third of hospitalized patients with risk factors for DVT received appropriate prophylactic measures. Without preventative treatment, up to 60 percent of patients undergoing total hip replacement surgery may develop a DVT. Symptoms of DVT include pain, tenderness, swelling or discoloration of the affected area and skin that is warm to the touch. As many as half of all cases produce minimal symptoms or are completely "silent."

A major complication from DVT is the development of pulmonary embolism (PE). This condition occurs when the blood clot from the lower extremity breaks loose from the wall of the vein and travels to the lungs, blocking the pulmonary artery or one of its branches. Patients with PE may show signs of shortness of breath, chest pain, rapid pulse, sweating, or bloody cough. Of those patients who develop PE, up to 200,000 will die each year.

By determining a patient's risk factors and providing appropriate prophylactic measures, the risk of DVT/PE is greatly reduced. In fact, the chances of a patient developing a PE with appropriate prophylaxis are reduced to less than 1%.

In order to provide the best quality care to the patients at Barnes-Jewish West County Hospital, the Pharmacy and Therapeutics and Medical Executive Committees have devised an Inpatient DVT Prophylaxis Assessment/Order Form in order to assist in the risk determination and therapy regimen for each specific patient. **Beginning on September 5, 2006, the order form will be included in the patient's admission packet and completed upon admission. The physician should review the patient's history in order to determine the applicable risk factors for that patient. He/she will then order the appropriate form of chemo- and mechanical prophylaxis.** The physician also has the option of ordering warfarin for those patients requiring longer prophylactic therapy. If the assessment/order form is not completed by the physician within 24 hours of admission, there will be a reminder placed in the front of the chart to ensure that DVT prophylaxis orders are received.

Figure 8.4. DVT: The road to prevention.

Conclusion

There can be no question that focusing on the prevention of DVT and PE is the "right" thing to do for the patient. Development of a successful program is not effortless. However, the rewards will be evident almost immediately, including decreased patient length of stay, decreased hospitalization costs, dramatic reductions in readmissions due to DVT or PE, enhanced patient awareness and education, as well as many other tangible and intangible benefits to both the organization and the patient. The success of the program depends largely on the dedication of the staff implementing it. It also requires continuous education and reeducation for staff and new employees. Frequent literature searches may be needed to keep the program up-to-date with new therapies or recommendations. The best way to ensure that a DVT/PE prophylaxis program is successful is to engrain it into the culture of the organization. Nurses, pharmacists, physicians, and other key personnel throughout the organization should take leading roles in ensuring the program remains alive and effective.

References

1. Caprini JA. Thrombosis risk assessment as a guide to quality patient care. *Dis Mon* 2005;70-78.
2. Prevention of venous thrombosis and pulmonary embolism. *Natl Inst Health Consen State* 1986;6(2):1-8.
3. Gross P, Weitz JI. Increasing awareness, optimizing prevention, and advancing treatment for VTE. American Society of Hematology. Available at: http://www.hematology.org/publications/hematologist/JA07/practicing.cfm.
4. Heit JA, Cohen AT, Anderson FA, et al. on behalf of the VTE Impact Assessment Group. Estimated annual number of incident and recurrent, non-fatal and fatal venous thromboembolism (VTE) events in the US. Poster #68. Presented at: 47th Annual Meeting and Exposition, American Society of Hematology; December 10-13, 2005; Atlanta, GA.
5. Gerotziafas GT, Samama MM. Prophylaxis of venous thromboembolism in medical patients. *Curr Opin Pulm Med* 2004;10:356-365.
6. Anderson FA Jr, Wheeler HB, Goldberg RJ, et al. A population-based perspective of the hospital incidence and case-fatality rates of deep vein thrombosis and pulmonary embolism. The Worcester DVT Study. *Arch Intern Med* 1991;151:933-938.
7. Heit JA. Venous thromboembolism epidemiology: implications for prevention and management. *Semin Thromb Hemost* 2002;28(suppl 2):3-13.
8. White RH. The epidemiology of venous thromboembolism. *Circulation* 2003;107:14-18.

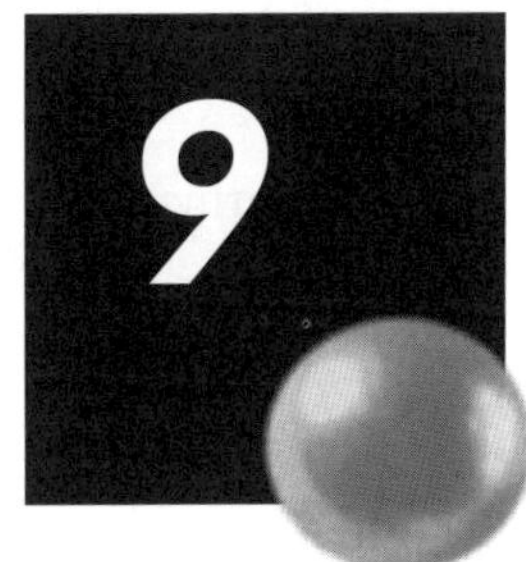

Clinical Communication: Is Your Staff Dialed In?

Rachel Hroncich

Background and Introduction

As clinical coordinator at Presbyterian Healthcare Services (PHS), I was given the somewhat daunting task of improving the way clinical communication was shared with the pharmacist staff at two of our hospitals in Albuquerque, New Mexico. As the largest health system in New Mexico, PHS employs over 75 pharmacists across the state, with the majority in our two Albuquerque facilities. These community hospitals have a combined total of 600 beds with almost every specialty provided, short of trauma and burn units. Most pharmacists are decentralized throughout the facilities, thanks to the continued support of our Pharmacy Department by our Administration. At PHS, we make no differentiation between "clinical" and "non-clinical" staff; every pharmacist is expected to function in both clinical and operational roles. Therefore, we faced the challenge of communicating clinical initiatives and education to pharmacists working at multiple sites, in multiple areas, on shifts occurring 24 hours a day.

When I assumed the clinical coordinator role, the method of clinical communication in existence was a 10-minute block at the end of the regular monthly operational staff meeting, where attendance included pharmacists and technicians (if they were scheduled to work that day and if they weren't too busy to leave their areas). Not an ideal communication situation for a new clinical coordinator with big clinical plans, the success of which depended upon understanding and acceptance by the staff pharmacists.

Clinical Conference: Identifying and Triaging the Obstacles

At first I tried to force my clinical initiatives into the staff meeting. The result was that the meeting expanded from its normal 45 minutes to about 1 hour and 15 minutes. This was far from ideal for staff with direct patient care responsibilities piling up in their absence. And because new clinical information was being presented, the pharmacists had many questions that were being rushed for the sake of time. It also left little room for staff to bring new ideas or concerns to the table. Additionally, the technician staff was being forced to sit through clinical information that did not necessarily apply to them.

Faced with this challenge, I redesigned the process of clinical communication. My first step was to meet with the Director of Pharmacy and the Operations Manager (who was in charge of the monthly staff meeting). Luckily, all were in agreement that the staff meeting was geared towards operations and not the best forum for disseminating clinical information. I proposed a separate pharmacist meeting that was only geared toward clinical information. The managers were slightly skeptical about the pharmacists attending "another meeting." This was a valid point of concern. To address this, we made the following three commitments: 1) Call for agenda topics from the staff to address any of their clinical requests, 2) make the meeting easy to participate in, and 3) request regular feedback from the staff regarding the usefulness of the meeting.

The first point is critical to gaining staff buy-in. The goal is to involve the pharmacists so they feel this is their meeting—a venue to explore clinical advancement. To that end, I sent out a request for agenda items. In the beginning, I received very little response. This was likely due to the fact that the staff was not sure what to expect from the meeting. However, after the first couple of meetings, pharmacists began submitting topics for discussion. They could choose to present the information themselves, or they could submit topics for me to address as clinical coordinator.

The agenda (Fig. 9.1) has a general format, incorporating those items offered by the pharmacists. The first section is always a "Reminders" section. This is an opportunity to reiterate and update the staff on clinical initiatives that have been recently rolled-out. It also provides a venue for the pharmacists to provide feedback regarding current initiatives. The next section is "Clinical News." This section includes everything from new clinical initiatives, Pharmacy & Therapeutics Committee (P&T) updates, and pharmacist-suggested topics. The last section, "Clinical Roundtable," is an open-call for discussion of any subject by any pharmacist.

When you have facilities that are staffed 24 hours per day with pharmacists working various shifts and days at multiple facilities, requiring attendance is not an option. On the other hand, assuming the information being shared is important, the opportunity and incentive to participate must be made available to all. The following accommodations are made to make the meetings as accessible as possible: 1) the meeting is held three times each month, twice at our larger facility and once at the smaller facility, 2) a teleconference line is arranged for pharmacists to dial-in from a remote location (e.g., the pediatric or operating room pharmacy satellites), and 3) pharmacists that dial in on their day off are compensated with 1 hour of pay at their normal pay rate. In addition, detailed minutes (including attachments) are sent out to all pharmacists via e-mail within 1 week of the meetings.

Some may argue that repeating the same meeting three times is not the best use of a clinical coordinator's time. However, if it takes three 1-hour meetings per month to be successful at a number of clinical initiatives, this is a small amount of time compared to the time wasted on ineffectively rolling out clinical initiatives that ultimately fail due to a lack of communication. It also gives the staff some face time with a member of the management team, which occurs less frequently these days as more initiatives (and thus, more work) become mandated by regulatory agencies.

Soliciting feedback and input from the pharmacists is a way to improve the meeting attendance, as well as provide an opportunity for the staff to become involved in management decision-making. The agenda always includes items that originate from the clinical coordinator, but also items that come from the staff. Pharmacists may call or email agenda topics. They may also suggest future agenda items on the meeting evaluation form (Fig. 9.2).

The meeting evaluation tool serves multiple purposes: 1) to ensure that the staff understands the information presented as it pertains to them, 2) to assess management's expectations

PRESBYTERIAN

Date: April 2008

Where: Pharm. Conference Room
I-25 and Kaseman

Presbyterian Healthcare Services - Pharmacy Department

Clinical Conference

** A G E N D A **

Rules: Excuse yourself if answering your Spectralink, share comments with the entire group, and stick to the topic.

Items:

Reminders

> Extended Infusion Beta-lactams - Feedback

> LMX, Recothrom

> Lovenox MUE - Feedback

Clinical News

> Pneumovax Orders: May 20th

> Coagucheck competency

> Dangerous Abbreviations: Erica

> Hycotuss - Hycodan substitution

> CNM Newsletter

> New adult TPN form: May 1st

> Alcohol dispensing

Clinical Round Table

> Successes

Notes:

Don't Forget to Complete a Meeting Evaluation!

Figure 9.1. Clinical conference agenda.

Pharmacy Clinical Conference
Post-Meeting Survey – April 2008

1. **Overall, did this meeting increase your knowledge of Pharmacy Clinical Services Initiatives?**

7 Definitely	6	5	4	3	2	1 Not at all

2. **Did this presentation provide new knowledge that will help you in your daily practice?**

7 Definitely	6	5	4	3	2	1 Not at all

3. **Overall, was today's meeting an effective use of your time?**

7 Very Effective	6	5	4	3	2	1 A Total Waste

4. **Did today's meeting increase your understanding of Pharmacy Administration's clinical expectations?**

7 Definitely	6	5	4	3	2	1 Not at all

5. **What are one or two of the most positive outcomes or events from today's meeting?**

6. **How could the meeting have been improved?**

7. **Future Agenda Item?**

Figure 9.2. Meeting evaluation.

of them as it relates to the items presented, 3) to comment on the high and low points of the meeting, 4) to suggest improvements to the meeting, and 4) to suggest topics for the next meeting. Every pharmacist is asked to complete an evaluation form before leaving the meeting. If you ask for input, you must be prepared to address the input in a constructive and meaningful way. If this does not occur, the staff may feel their input is not valued and will disengage from the process.

Expectations of the Staff

As with any profession, there is a spectrum of engagement by individual pharmacists in management-directed activities. Because the information being presented at the clinical conference is deemed worthy of presenting, it should also be viewed as important enough that all pharmacists understand what is being presented each month. Therefore, all pharmacists are required to participate in one way or another. Pharmacists that are unable to attend or dial-in are expected to send an acknowledgement of the minutes via e-mail to the clinical coordinator. Monthly participation is recorded and reviewed as part of pharmacist annual evaluations. Documentation is also made with regards to those pharmacists who submit and present agenda items so that this behavior can be acknowledged and encouraged as part of annual evaluations.

Benefits

Several positive outcomes have been observed since the inception of clinical conference at our facility in 2006. First, the ease with which clinical initiatives are rolled-out across the two facilities has increased exponentially. If a new clinical project is in the works, I bring it up as an FYI one month and then roll it out at the next meeting, giving the pharmacists more than one opportunity to hear about it before the initiative begins. If something is going to be on the next P&T agenda, I will use the clinical conference to solicit feedback from the pharmacists before the item makes it to the P&T agenda. Many times, the pharmacists identify issues not noted previously.

Clinical conference also provides a forum for sharing new clinical information. For example, when the Food and Drug Administration (FDA) alerted the healthcare community of the potential risks with erythropoiesis-stimulating agents (ESAs), clinical conference was a great venue for discussing the impact these alerts have on our patients and for brainstorming how best to address these alerts. Pharmacists also bring copies of journal articles to share with the rest of the staff regarding research they feel the group would benefit from knowing. Additionally, the pharmacists will share brief clinical pearls they have recently addressed in their practice area so that the entire group can benefit. This clinical input from the staff has helped to motivate all pharmacists to stay on top of the latest medical literature, as well as look for ways to improve clinical outcomes as a health system.

The required participation also helps to foster accountability. Pharmacists can no longer say "I didn't know about that new medication use evaluation"; if it was presented at clinical conference, they are expected to know about it. In the beginning, it took some one-on-one counseling to help those pharmacists understand the new expectation of participation in clinical conference. However, this was self-limiting as most employees would rather participate than answer questions from their clinical coordinator as to why they did not know about a new process. As previously discussed, if participation is required, it is important to make it as easy as possible to participate. Since reading the minutes and acknowledging them via an e-mail to the clinical coordinator counts as participation, no one has an excuse not to participate.

Another benefit of clinical conference is that it significantly decreased the time of the monthly operational staff meetings. This was deemed a great advantage by the pharmacist and technician staffs, as well as the operations manager. The staff meetings returned to 45 minutes in length, a time that is much more reasonable for staff with direct patient care responsibilities.

Perhaps one of the most important outcomes of the clinical conference was the opportunity for a large pharmacist staff to interact on a clinical level. If the staff did not gain some benefit from getting together as a group, they could choose just to read the electronic minutes. I believe this peer interaction may be the main reason that attendance at the actual meeting consistently ranges between 75-90% of the staff who is working that day. Additionally, at the end of each meeting, each pharmacist shares one intervention he or she made recently that positively impacted patient care. This provides each pharmacist the opportunity to receive recognition from their peers for a job well done. They also reflect on what they do, as a group, to improve patient outcomes.

An unexpected benefit of clinical conference was easy documentation of the dissemination of clinical information to the pharmacists. This came in handy during a recent Joint Commission (JC) survey. When asked by a surveyor, "How do your pharmacists learn about new drugs that are added to the formulary?" I was able to pull out the clinical conference minutes, as well as the documentation of the pharmacists' acknowledgement of the minutes. This was viewed favorably by the surveyor.

Conclusion

Getting a large, multi-site pharmacist staff to engage in clinical communication is not an easy task. But if management is committed to putting forth the effort to make the communication easily accessible and beneficial to the staff, many obstacles can be overcome. By encouraging feedback and outlining pharmacist expectations, the staff can be empowered to actively participate and contribute. Success in implementing new initiatives can be attributed to the success of the clinical conference meetings.

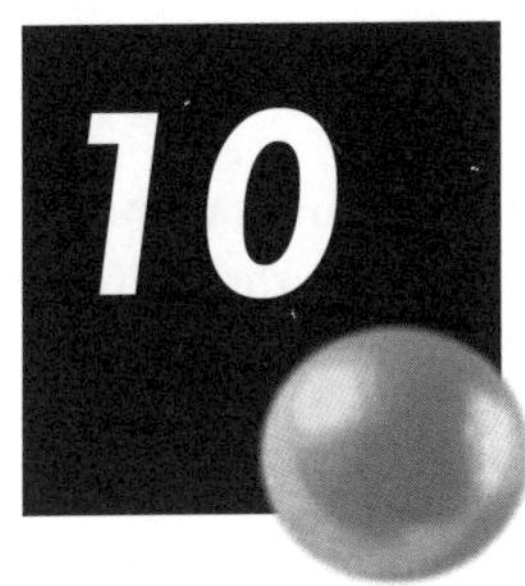

Intervention Follow-Through: Is IT Being Done?

Georgeanne Lemanowicz

Hospital

Southwest General Health Center is a private, not-for-profit, 354-bed facility located in Middleburg Heights, Ohio. The hospital serves southwestern Cuyahoga, eastern Lorain and northern Medina counties. Founded in 1920, Southwest General has a deep commitment to providing a healthy future for its patients, families, and communities.

The health center offers a full range of services including a Level III trauma center, cardiovascular surgery, three urgent care centers, a behavioral health facility, geriatric assessment and elder evaluation program, a pharmacist-managed Coumadin clinic, home health, maternity services, orthopedic surgery, orthopedic joint and spine skilled unit, an acute rehabilitation unit, and a residential hospice. Southwest General's mission statement is: *Health is our Business; Quality is our Focus; Compassion is our Way.*

Background

Pharmacist interventions occur every hour of every day, but unfortunately, are not all recorded. As part of pharmacists daily duties not only are they preventing prescribing errors, but the pharmacists provide cognitive services, including therapeutic drug monitoring, drug-use review, patient and physician education, and disease management.[1,2,3] There have been many studies showing the value of the pharmacist, not only saving costs for their institutions, but more importantly, protecting and safeguarding the patient. The Joint Commission of Accreditation of Healthcare Organizations (JCAHO) requires that all medications are reviewed by a pharmacist before administration and emphasizes the importance of pharmacists' documentation of outcomes of their interventions.[4] The problem has been, and continues to be, finding a quick and easy method to assist the pharmacist in keeping track of their interventions. Southwest General Health Center uses their pharmacy order entry system to document, track, and report pharmacist interventions.

The pharmacy department has 19.5 pharmacist full-time employees (FTEs) in clinical or dispensing roles. It is the responsibility of the QA pharmacist to analyze and report pharmacist interventions, not only to the staff and pharmacy management, but also to various committees throughout the institution. The information is validation of the positive impact the pharmacy department has on patient care. The pharmacy department had been documenting interventions using Cerner Classic since 1996. The average number of pharmacist interventions per month in 2005 was 210. The monthly average number of intervention increased to 300 through July of 2006. The pharmacy converted to Cerner Millennium Pharmnet in August of 2006. Due to the post conversion learning curve, the documentation of interventions suffered. But in January 2007, the interventions climbed close to pre-conversion numbers. And in 2007, the monthly average number of interventions was 313. The categories for the majority of the interventions documented by the pharmacy department documents are: dose adjustments, pharmacokinetics, laboratory value and medication monitoring, formulary conversions, medication history interventions and clarifications, optimizing administration route, optimizing medication durations, order clarifications, and patient counseling/teaching interventions.

The institution wanted mechanisms in place to assist the pharmacists in following through on incomplete interventions. These incomplete interventions could be due to several factors, including pending laboratory levels and waiting on physicians, nursing, family members, or outpatient pharmacies to return phone calls and pages. This usually occurs when the problem needs to be carried over from shift to shift, if the resolution could not be completed while that pharmacist was on duty. Verification processes are needed not only to ensure that interventions are documented but that pharmacists start the documentation process for incomplete interventions and that interventions are completed and the outcome of the interventions are captured. The Southwest General pharmacy department decided that one of the department's goals was to increase the number of interventions recorded. The department also was looking for a process that would assist in completing the interventions in a timely manner.

Intervention

Southwest General pharmacy department wanted to use technology to its advantage to ensure that unresolved interventions were being acted upon. The department's technology includes MedSelect's InterChange product as its physician order management system and Cerner's Millennium computer system. The InterChange system prioritizes the incoming physicians' orders from the nursing units, links the orders to the patients, has a user friendly retrieval system, and the ability to fax orders back to the nursing units. Two useful features are the ability to annotate the orders and place orders on hold. The pharmacy department wanted to use all resources available to alert the parties involved that there were medication orders that needed further attention. The department developed several different procedures to assist in the process.

The first method was to annotate on the physician's order sheets in the InterChange system with the problem, and the current action plan. The annotated order is faxed to the nursing unit using the fax back feature on InterChange so that the nurse is notified of the problem. The order is then put on hold until it is resolved. The department has the hold feature defaulted to a 2-hour hold, which can be modified at the pharmacist's discretion. One advantage of the hold feature is that when the time period has expired, the order will appear in the order queue as the next available order, which serves as a reminder to the pharmacist that the problem still has not been resolved. Another positive of the hold queue is each order has the patient's name clearly visible so that any pharmacist at a computer terminal has a visual cue of the problem order when the physician or nurse calls back. The pharmacist can quickly retrieve the order without having to look around for a paper record.

Name	Discharge DT/TM	Orig Order DT/TM	Order Sentence
		2/15/2008 20:26:38	TNF - A PROBLEM IRON 500MG 1 EA Non Formulary ORAL PROTOCOL
		2/15/2008 23:18:59	TNF - A PROBLEM: SULFASALAZINE 1 EA Non Formulary ORAL PROTOCOL
			TNF - A PROBLEM: VITAMIN B12 SHOT 1 EA Non Formulary IM PROTOCOL
		2/15/2008 01:58:52	TNF - A PROBLEM: XANAX ON MED REC SHEET 1 EA Non Formulary NONE PROTOCOL
		2/15/2008 23:24:32	TNF - A PROBLEM: HUMALOG SLIDE SCALE ON MED REC SHEET 1 EA Non Formulary NONE PROTOCOL
		2/15/2008 07:34:29	TNF - A PROBLEMS-SOD CHLORIDE 5% & PELEVANS 1 EA Non Formulary ORAL PROTOCOL
		2/15/2008 21:53:17	TNF - A PROBLEM XALATAN FREQUENCY 1 EA Non Formulary OPH PROTOCOL
			TNF - A PROBLEM ZYVOX, NEED ID APPROVAL 1 EA Non Formulary ORAL PROTOCOL
		2/15/2008 12:10:02	TNF - A PROBLEM: KADIAN 1 EA Non Formulary ORAL PROTOCOL
		2/15/2008 19:24:11	TNF - A PROBLEM: LO-ESTRIN-24 1 EA Non Formulary ORAL PROTOCOL
		2/14/2008 02:32:34	TNF - A PROBLEM WITH ISOSORBIDE 1 EA Non Formulary ORAL PROTOCOL

Figure 10.1. Problem order report.

A process that is used by the institution to increase communication and awareness is a method in which the problem medication orders are entered into the Millennium Pharm-Net computer system. Any order that needs clarification is entered using a non-formulary pathway. It is entered as "A Problem" and then the drug name. The frequency is listed as protocol. This way, if a Computer Generated Medication Administration Record (CMAR) prints during the time the order is waiting for clarification, the problem medication order will appear as the first order on the CMAR because the CMAR is in alphabetical order. The "A Problem" orders serve as a reminder to the staff that there is a problem with the medication, and they can potentially assist in the clarification process. This is especially helpful with admission orders because a MAR is printed after the admission orders are entered in the system and the nurse may notice the entry on the MAR before seeing the faxed back order. Often times, the nurse has contact with the physician and can clarify the order before pharmacy has a chance to call the physician. We also use the "A Problem" to designate medications from home that need to be identified before they can be used in the institution. The pharmacy department prints a report daily at 7:00 AM of the list of the current problem orders (Fig. 10.1). The list can also be printed by the clinical/decentralized pharmacists anywhere in the hospital so they can clarify any outstanding orders on their units.

The next process involves the actual interventions themselves. Millennium PowerChart gives the department the ability to not only capture completed intervention but pending interventions as well. The pharmacy department has a generic intervention document that is used as a template for the interventions (Fig. 10.2). The intervention form has some mandatory fields and other optional fields. Intervention type is one of the mandatory fields. To make the entry process fast and painless for the pharmacy staff, the form has most of the usual types of interventions listed so the pharmacy can quickly select the type of intervention. This includes adverse drug event reporting, doses that are too high and too low, drug information questions, drug interactions, formulary conversions, optimizing administration route, order clarification, patient counseling, pharmacokinetic consults, therapeutic duplications, and unnecessary medication orders. The other mandatory fields include person initiating the intervention, clinical importance of the intervention, prescriber response, intervention outcome, and actual time spent on the intervention. All the mandatory fields have the common elements listed to speed up completion of the intervention. The optional fields include the associated orders, pharmacoeconomic impact, and the physician's name. The pharmacists usually type a short explanation, but it is not required.

Clinical Interventions

*Intervention Type

○ Adverse drug event	○ Dose too low	○ Drug, lab interaction	○ Optimize formulation	○ Pharmacokinetic consult
○ Dose too high	○ Drug information question	○ Formulary conversion	○ Optimize frequency	○ Therapeutic duplication
○ Dose too high-age	○ Drug, disease interaction	○ Medication history	○ Optimize monitoring	○ Unnecessary order
○ Dose too high-renal	○ Drug, drug interaction	○ Optimize administration route	○ Order clarification	○ Untreated indication
○ Dose too high-weight	○ Drug, food interaction	○ Optimize duration	○ Patient counseling	○ Other:

Associated Order(s)

*Initiated By

○ Nurse
○ Pharmacist
○ Physician
○ Other:

*Clinical Importance

○ Potentially severe
○ Potentially major
○ Potentially minor
○ Little or no clinical importance
○ Other:

Severe - Fatal or severe error/life threatening

Major - Affect organ function or quality of life

Minor - Care to more acceptable level

*Prescriber Response

○ Accepted
○ Corrected prior to contact
○ Modified
○ No response
○ Not accepted
○ Patient dismissed before response
○ Pending
○ Other:

Prescriber

Pharmacoeconomic Impact

○ < $5.00	○ $100.01 - $250.00
○ $5.01 - $15.00	○ $250.01 - $500.00
○ $15.01 - $25.00	○ $500.01 - $1000.00
○ $25.01 - $50.00	○ > $1000.00
○ $50.01 - $100.00	

*Patient Clinical Outcome

○ Not applicable
○ Avoided potential risk
○ Negative outcome from recommendation
○ No change from recommendation
○ Patient responded to recommendation
○ Pending
○ Unknown
○ Other:

*Pharmacist Intervention Time

○ < 1 Minute	○ 16-30 Minutes
○ 1-5 Minutes	○ > 30 Minutes
○ 6-15 Minutes	

Additional Information

Figure 10.2. Clinical interventions report.

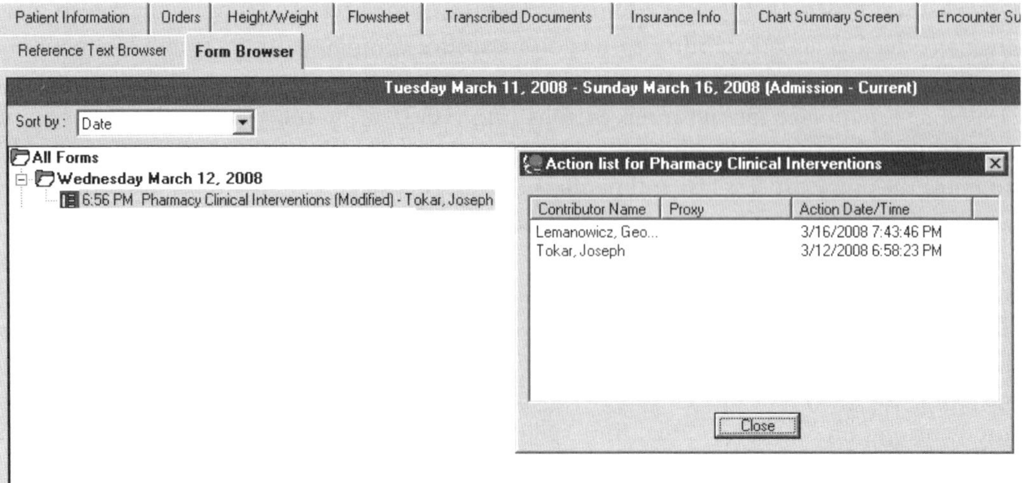

Figure 10.3. Intervention log.

```
Time: 08:50 am                PHARMACY PENDING INTERVENTION REPORT                Page: 1
-----------------------------------------------------------------------------------------

2W  W272-01  [last name, first name]          Fin nbr:

          Prescriber Response: Pending

               Intervention Type: Other: ANTIBIOTIC SURVEILLANCE.

               Additional Info: CALLED TO CHECK INDICATION. NO CULTURES ORDERED AT THIS TIME

3W  W364-02  [last name, first name]          Fin nbr:

          Prescriber Response: Pending

               Intervention Type: Medication history

               Additional Info: Called concering allergies to pain meds and antibiotics. RN to interview patient


Time: 07:21 am                PHARMACY PENDING INTERVENTION REPORT                Page: 1
-----------------------------------------------------------------------------------------

2N  N210-01  [last name, first name]          Fin nbr: 1

          Prescriber Response: Accepted

               Intervention Type: Pharmacokinetic consult

               Additional Info: TOBRAMYCIN MONITORING

2N  N246-01  [last name, first name]          Fin nbr:

          Prescriber Response: Pending

               Intervention Type: Medication history

               Additional Info: CALLED TO CLARIFY THREE MEDS.  RN WILL CALL FAMILY.WROTE ORDER FOR STOOL SOFTEN


2N  N251-02  [last name, first name]          Fin nbr: 4

          Prescriber Response: Corrected prior to c

               Intervention Type: Other: one dose of avelox sent until md can be called
```

Figure 10.4. Pharmacy pending intervention report.

Once the interventions are completed, the pharmacist can either chart the intervention or save it. Charting the intervention completes it, whereas saving the intervention leaves it in process or pending. The pharmacy department took advantage of the ability to save or chart the orders. If the intervention was not complete the pharmacists were instructed to save the intervention instead of completing it. Any intervention that is saved, or if pending is selected for the outcome or physician response, will be included in the pending intervention reports. Although it is highly encouraged to save all pending interventions, it is most helpful to enter pending interventions in which follow up will occur over several days like pharmacokinetics or lab values that are pending. Millennium PowerChart has a nice documentation trail for the interventions. Anyone can view not only the intervention but who charted what action (Fig. 10.3). A report is generated on a daily basis that lists all the pending interventions (Fig. 10.4). This report can be reviewed any where in the institution by the pharmacists, nurses, and physicians.

The hospital strives to increase communication among caregivers and between patients and caregivers. We participate in the national patient advocacy program, SPEAK UP, encouraging patients to take an active role in their care. Among staff, we have instituted several initiatives, including order read back on all telephone orders. This process is an excellent tool to verify that the order is heard correctly. Another method of improving department to department communication is the introduction of the Vocera system. Several departments in the hospital are using this quick and effective voice recognition communication system, including the emergency department and the pharmacy. This system ensures immediate contact between staff members and between departments. As with the intervention process, the hospital uses Cerner Millennium in many ways to increase the information available to nurses and physicians. We are using Millennium PowerChart, whereby all necessary patient information, including medications, meds reconciliation process, diet orders, radiology reports, lab values, and emergency department vitals are available to appropriate staff members and physicians.

Conclusion

The Southwest General Health Center pharmacy department is using the technology at its disposal to try to assist the pharmacist in not only documentation of interventions but in completing interventions in a timely manner. Documentation of interventions is vital in providing hospital administration with justification that pharmacists provide an integral role in improving overall patient care.[5] Southwest General's pharmacist interventions are steadily increasing. Providing routine feedback to pharmacists about the types of interventions that they have documented and their performance relative to others may serve as an incentive as well. [6] At Southwest General, there is a push for the pharmacists to document their interventions because it is believed that the numbers are still under reported. An incentive to increase documentation of interventions is the modification of the pharmacists' performance evaluations to include each pharmacist's statistical data concerning interventions. Their individual performance has a partial impact on their annual performance-based salary increase. Southwest's technology is being used effectively to assist not only in increasing communication between the pharmacists and nurses of the problem medication orders/interventions that need to be completed but in assisting in the tabulation of the interventions.

References

1. Jaber LA, Halapy H, Fernet M. Evaluation of a pharmaceutical care model on diabetes management. *Ann Pharmacother* 1996;30:294-5.
2. Lee YP, Schommer JC. Effect of pharmacist managed anticoagulation clinic on Warfarin related hospital readmission. *Am J Health-Syst Pharm* 1996;53:1580-3.
3. Lippy EA, Laub JJ. Economic and clinical impact of a pharmacy based antihypertensive replacement program in primary care. *Am J Health-Syst Pharm* 1997:54:2079-83.
4. Accreditation Manual for Hospital.Chicago: Joint Commission on Accreditation of Health Care Organizations, 1988.
5. Heslett TM, Kay BG, Weissfellner H. Documenting concurrent clinical pharmacy interventions. *Hosp Pharm* 1990;25:
6. Chin JM, Muller PJ, Lucarelli DC. A pharmacy intervention program. Recognizing pharmacy's contribution to improving patient care. *Hosp Pharm* 1995;30(2):120,123-6,129-30.

Documenting Interventions: A Practice of the Past

E. Thomas Carey

Introduction and Institution

SwedishAmerican Hospital is a 357-bed community teaching hospital located in Rockford, Illinois. Incorporating an academic model of providing clinical pharmacist services into a community hospital, SwedishAmerican Hospital has provided extensive clinical pharmacy services since 1992. Currently, 11 pharmacists provide clinical services to all inpatient areas in addition to the operating room, outpatient oncology clinic, and the emergency department. In addition to typical functions and programs, the clinical pharmacists are members of the trauma, stroke, and cardiac arrest teams. They provide training and didactic lectures to pharmacy students from multiple pharmacy schools, provide community education through local media outlets, and participate in several national and international clinical trials.

Though supported in concept by organizations such as The Joint Commission, the Leap Frog Group, and the Institute of Medicine, pharmacy leaders are challenged to justify the impact of clinical pharmacists to health system administrators. Financially justifying the expense of clinical pharmacists traditionally has been and continues to be challenging for pharmacy leadership. Cost saving initiatives are often insufficient to offset the high cost of pharmacist salaries. Typically, documentation of interventions performed by clinical pharmacists is commonly used to further qualify the value provided by clinical pharmacists. However, this accepted concept has several shortcomings. This chapter describes how coordination of activities and collectively quantifying their financial impact has negated the need for clinical pharmacists to document interventions using traditional models.

Shortcomings of Traditional Model

Like most clinical pharmacists, the staff at SwedishAmerican Hospital documented interventions as part of their regular functions. The information technology tool used at SwedishAmerican Hospital is Meditech. The software has pre-built spreadsheets to document multiple types of interventions such as:

- Intravenous to oral (IV to PO dosing) dosage form conversion
- Renal dosing
- Pharmacokinetic monitoring

- Adverse drug reaction identification
- Medication error identification
- Antibiotic selection and monitoring

The culmination of these interventions were then collected and summarized. Ultimately, the data was used to highlight the workload of each clinical pharmacist. However, though the actual number of documented interventions appeared high, it did not seem to correlate with the actual workload. As such, we conducted a 12-week review of the process for documenting interventions. The goal of the review was to compare the number of interventions documented

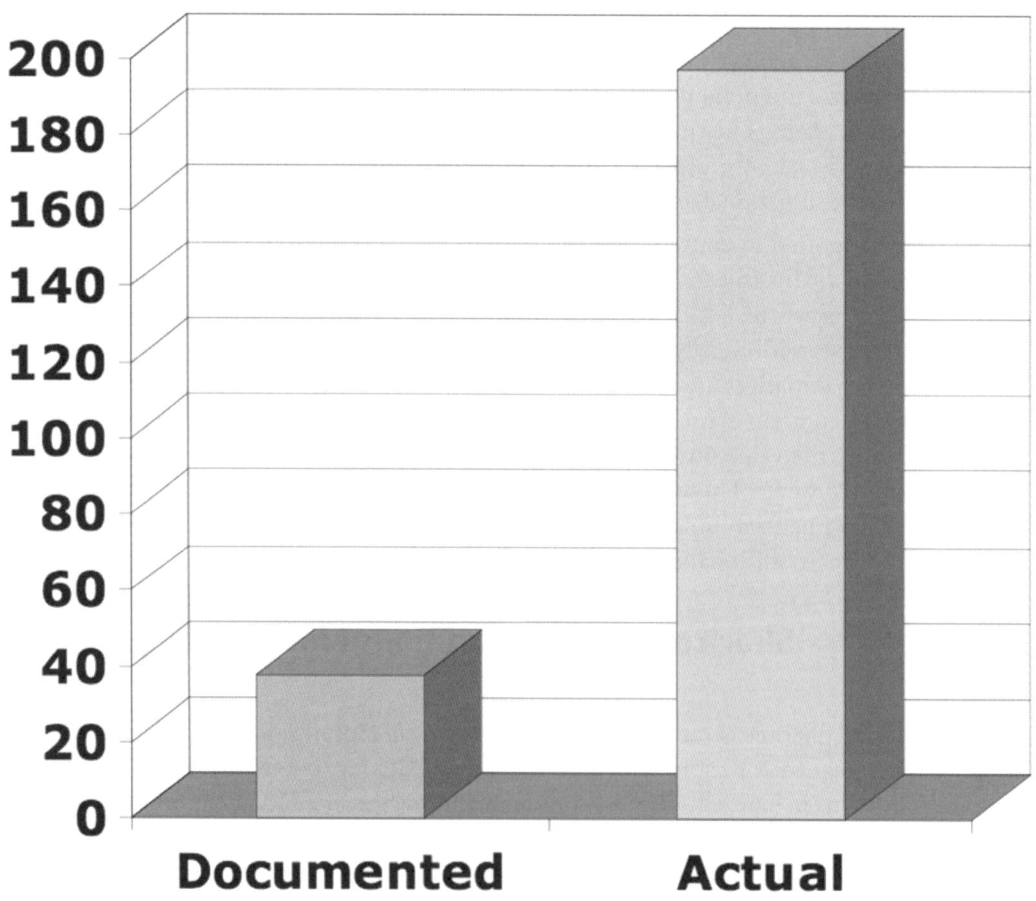

Figure 11.1. Actual versus documented interventions by clinical pharmacists each month.

Table 11.1. Advantages and Disadvantages of Homegrown vs. Commercial Systems

	Advantages	Disadvantages
Homegrown Systems	Can be institution-specific	Internal programming time
	Interventions can be patient-specific	No external benchmarks for comparison
	Low cost	
Commercial Systems	Can benchmark to other institutions	Often relies on "soft dollars"
	Provides extensive reporting capabilities	Lack of integration to internal systems
		Lacks standardization between products
		High cost

when the emphasis was not stressed to quantifying every potential intervention. The net result showed a disconnect between the two processes (Fig. 11.1).

The result of the trial demonstrated two issues. First, although the clinical pharmacists documented many interventions, it was usually for "high ticket" items, such as IV to PO conversions, renal dosing, and pharmacokinetic monitoring. Although these clinical initiatives are significant, they only comprised a minority of interventions. Medication information questions, chart reviews when no interventions were made, in-services, and meetings were not documented. The clinical pharmacists spent a great deal of time in these areas, but may not have had a significant result each time the intervention or interaction occurred. Regardless, by not documenting these areas, the clinical pharmacists were not providing actual pictures of their workloads.

The second issue that was identified through the review was the amount of time spent to document all interventions. Each clinical pharmacist spent an average of 83 minutes per day documenting interventions. Although the database is pre-built and accessible, a significant proportion of time is required to document all interventions.

There are multiple options available to document interventions. Homegrown technologies include internal databases using current information systems tools or Microsoft Office software such as Microsoft Excel or Access. Commercial solutions include CliniTrend®, Quantifi®, CliniDoc®, Health Point Link®, and many others. Both have advantages and disadvantages in their utility (Table 11.1).

Table 11.2. Financial Impact of Clinical Pharmacist Interventions

Cost Reduction Initiatives

	FY04	FY05	FY06	FY07
Renal Dosing	22,922.63	25,838.00	41,536.95	$58,182
IV to Oral	5,701.00	13,313.00	11,662.05	$18,626
Total =	28,623.63	39,151.00	53,199.00	$76,808

Revenue Enhancement

	FY04	FY05	FY06	FY07
Pneumovax Program	$6,000	$6,000	$17,373.00	$42,978
OR Pharmacy Satellite	$819,681	$797,123	$823,963	$832,400
Total =	$825,681	$803,123	$841,336.00	$875,378.00
				$952,186.45

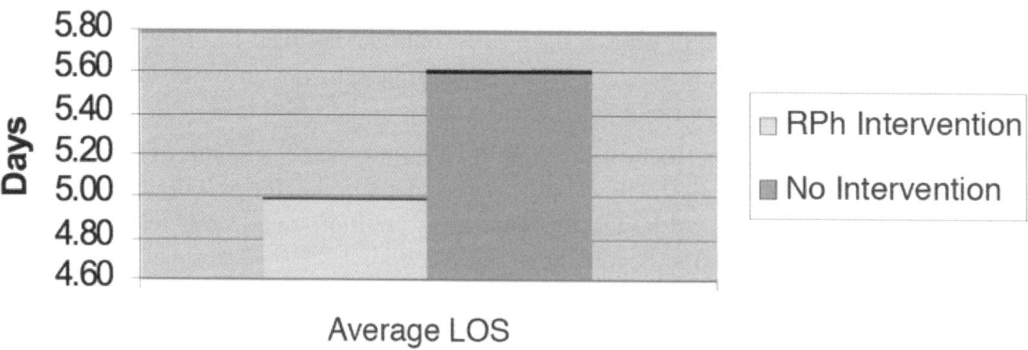

Figure 11.2. Length-of-stay (LOS) was directly correlated to clinical pharmacy intervention. No inventions increased patient LOS.

Table 11.3. Return on Investment for Clinical Pharmacists

	FY07
Clinical Pharmacist Salaries	$715,121.00
Cost Savings	$952,186.45
ROI =	**$1.33**

The Solution

The goal in moving forward was to be able to capture data pertaining to clinical pharmacist initiatives while minimizing the time required quantifying the activities. The initial step was to identify specific initiatives that provided significant clinical or financial implications. One example included renal dosing of medications. Using our current information system, clinical pharmacists "flag" the target medications. For example, after the pharmacist identifies the intervention, they enter the new order into the Meditech pharmacy information system. Concurrently, they enter a code into a pre-built field such as "renal dosing." Because this function is a component of their normal functions, they do not separately document interventions. Each predefined target medication is treated in the same manner.

At periodic intervals (i.e., monthly or quarterly), the sum of the interventions are downloaded into internally created spreadsheets. Each intervention is assigned a "cost savings" value. The value is based upon a combination of actual cost differences and data retrieved from published studies. For example, actual cost savings for renal dosing adjustments are determined from wholesaler acquisition costs. This is coupled with data from published literature, which has quantified average number of doses captured based on specific interventions. The data are then downloaded into a spreadsheet, which automates the financial impact of all clinical pharmacist interventions (Table 11.2).

Using the same "flagging" system, data can also be extracted to identify differences in length of stay. For example, with the Meditech Report Writer capabilities, patients discharged with a pneumonia diagnosis can be separated into two groups – those for whom a clinical pharmacist switched from an IV to an oral formulation and those patients for whom clinical pharmacists did not make similar interventions (Fig. 11.2).

All predefined target initiatives can be collected together to provide a net fiscal result of both cost savings and revenue enhancement initiatives. When balanced against the expenditure for pharmacist salaries, we can create a positive return on investment. As such, we have demonstrated that for every one dollar spent on a clinical pharmacist, the health system recognizes a cost savings or revenue enhancement of $1.33 (Table 11.3).

Conclusion

Pharmacy leaders are continually challenged to be able to justify the economic expenditure of clinical pharmacists. They are further challenged in that the primary mechanism to be able to do this is often inefficient. By using pre-existing software and targeting specific interventions, we have been able to demonstrate a positive return on investment while avoiding additional workload to our clinical pharmacist staff.

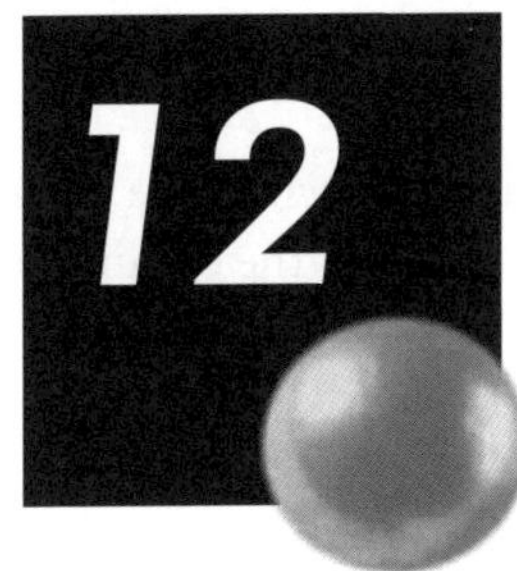

Today's Formulary Management

Tammy Cohen
Erin Sears

Background

Formulary management has become increasingly difficult in recent years for many reasons. The number of medications on the market continues to increase, and the individual agents have become more complex with a growing number of niche agents that have unique mechanisms of action. In turn, the number of single-agent drug classes has increased. Identifying a preferred agent in each drug class can be difficult, and it is more difficult to eliminate a whole class. Another factor that makes formulary management complicated is the increase in combination agents, and more importantly, combination agents consisting of strengths not available as individual components (e.g., BiDil). A third component is direct-to-consumer advertising. Patients now request specific products by name, which may or may not be the formulary agent of choice. Additionally, there is debate regarding the necessity of maintaining all home medication use during a hospital admission (e.g., statins). A final factor is patient use of alternative products and the lack of regulation associated with their use.

Institution

Baylor Health Care System (BHCS) has been challenged to streamline the formularies of its member institutions in hopes of creating a standardized approach across the system. Baylor is located in the Dallas- Fort Worth metroplex and consists of 13 hospitals, which include a large private teaching facility, two heart hospitals, a rehabilitation facility, a specialty hospital, and several community sites totaling over 3000 licensed beds. The current pharmacy and therapeutics (P&T) structure includes a system wide P&T Advisory Board and a P&T Committee at each individual site.

Formulary management strategies are based on clinical and financial opportunities. Drug classes are targeted if defined as high volume/low cost or high volume/high cost. Other medications evaluated for financial opportunities are those appearing in the top 50 drug spend report.

High Volume/Low Cost Medications

High volume agents are reviewed to reduce line items. This has been completed for multivitamins, renal vitamins, creams, ointments, insulins, and statins. Although this is not a direct cost savings initiative, standardizing these agents alleviates operational issues, such as the need to stock all agents in each automated dispensing cabinet and enter all agents into the computer order entry system.

High Volume/High Cost Medications

High volume/high cost drug classes are reviewed to reduce line items. The initial classes reviewed included anti-infectives, cardiac medications, statins, and insulins. Each review includes formulary recommendations and an implementation kit consisting of a detailed monograph, draft newsletter materials, conversion chart, and financial analysis, as appropriate. Follow-up includes a monthly report of key initiatives that shows market share and actual savings. Any issues that arise are addressed in the bi-weekly clinical liaison meeting.

Top Drug Spend Medications

The initial focus at BHCS was on the top agents on the drug spend report. A report is compiled monthly of the top 50 drug spend agents by site and rolled-up for the system. Various dosages are rolled into one line item (e.g., Levaquin of all strengths are reported as one line item, vaccines are reported as one line item, all insulins are reported as one item). Rolling up the various dosage forms allowed for a more accurate representation of drug spend. At BHCS, the top 10 drug spend line items equate to 28% of all drug spend. Each of the top 10 items was evaluated individually for opportunities. Intravenous to oral conversion programs, contract opportunities, and formulary status across all sites were evaluated and streamlined whenever possible.

A rolling 12 months of drug spend is reported monthly to account for seasonal variances. The reports are trended to identify early changes and to validate desired market share shifts. This data is then presented at the system P&T Advisory Board and the individual P&T Committees. The physician members have become increasingly engaged in the process and are readily able to identify where the most money is spent and participate in questioning, allowing for tighter control on contracts. For example, blood factors were being used more frequently at one facility in comparison to the other sites. The report demonstrated that a more in-depth look was needed to ensure clinical appropriateness. Additionally, when a conversion was completed for a given anti-infective class and purchases for the previously used product appeared, the physicians requested that the prescriber be identified to ensure contract compliance.

Conclusion

Formulary management is complex for a variety of reasons, and a multifaceted approach is necessary for its proper management. A combination of clinical and financial evaluations is needed to find opportunities to maximize operational ease, financial gain, and most importantly, clinical outcomes.

Part

3

Financial Management

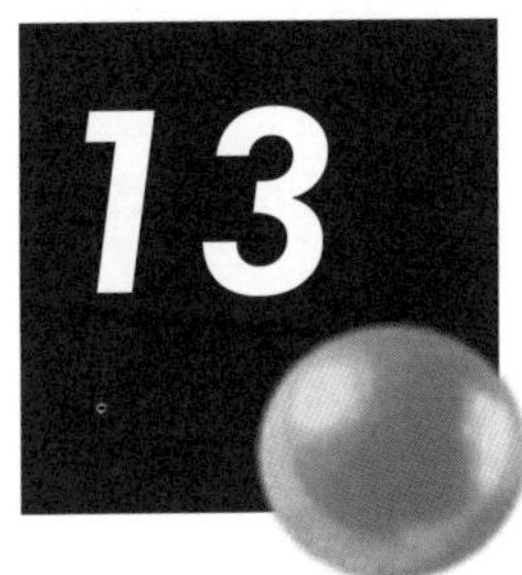

Reimbursement for Pharmaceuticals: I Know You're Bluffing

Anne T. Jarrett

Background and Introduction

Hospital pharmacists are considered to be an important part of the health care team, often rounding with physicians and other members. Pharmacists play an important role by routinely performing integral tasks, such as providing drug information, recommending appropriate drug therapy, monitoring its usage, reconciling medications, and ensuring that the right medicine gets to the right patient at the right time. However, there is one question that stumps most pharmacists: What is the reimbursement for drug X?

In today's healthcare environment, pharmacists are forced to acknowledge that health care is a business. Understanding reimbursement for pharmaceuticals is part of making the business successful. One would think that someone in another department, such as medical coding or medical records, should be responsible for this. However, the onus has been put on the pharmacy department to make sure they are using the right codes, keeping up with the frequent changes, and lastly, being aware of the amount of reimbursement received by the hospital. Reimbursement should be a part of formulary decisions and management, purchasing drugs, and negotiating contracts. The importance of cost effectiveness is not new. Reimbursement is just a part of that and has become increasingly more important every year.

Most hospital pharmacists need the following:

- Understanding of the process and policies of reimbursement
- Educational materials specifically targeted to pharmacists
- More non-clinical learning for pharmacists
- Role model to show reimbursement in action

Education for Hospital Pharmacists About Pharmaceutical Reimbursement

The ASHP Section of Pharmacy Practice Managers' Advisory Group (SAG) on Finance and Reimbursement created a resource on the ASHP website to provide information about pharmaceutical reimbursement. Even though the resource center has been available several years, many pharmacists are not aware of its existence. Pharmacists should navigate through the ASHP site to become familiar with pharmaceutical reimbursement.

The Resource Center

First, go to ASHP's website, which can be found at http://www.ashp.org

Then, go to "Resource Centers," on the bottom right of the Home page and choose "Pharmaceutical Reimbursement" from the drop-down menu. There you will see the home page of the resource center.

There are four major categories, entitled:

1. *What's New*
2. *Getting Started*
3. *Learn More*
4. *Tools for Practice*

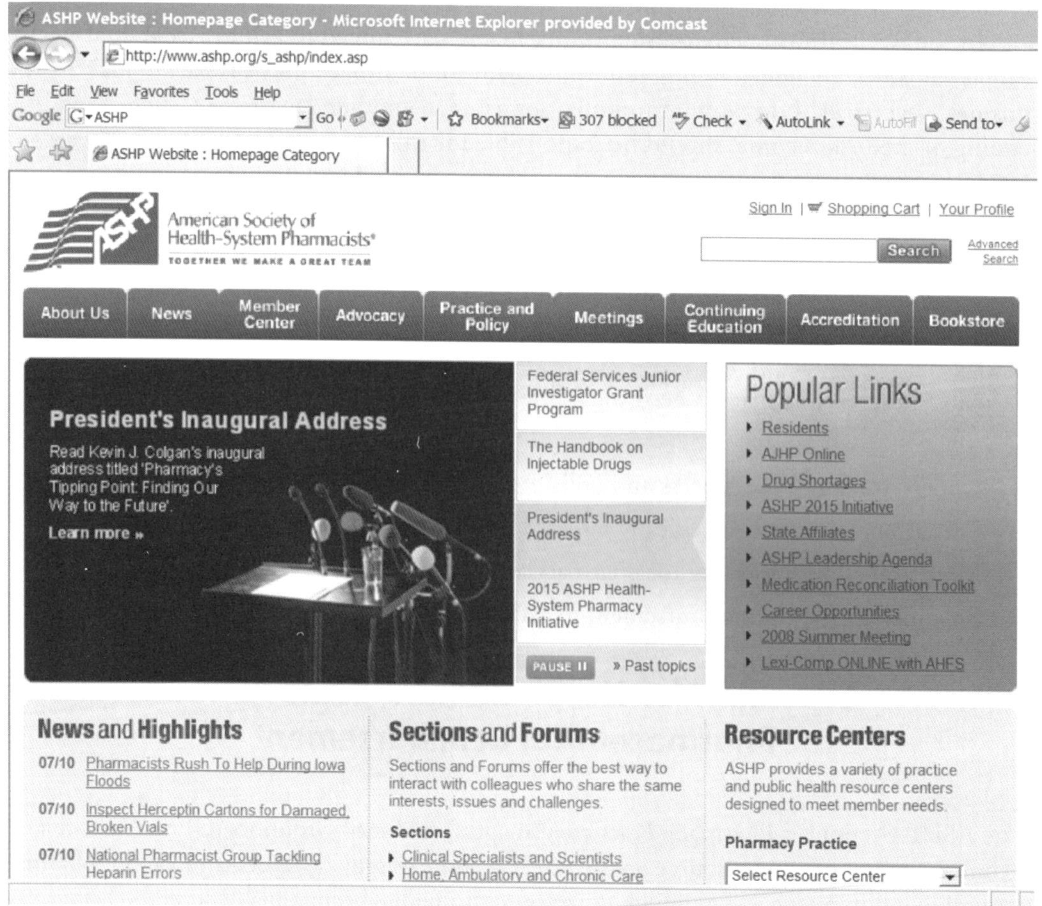

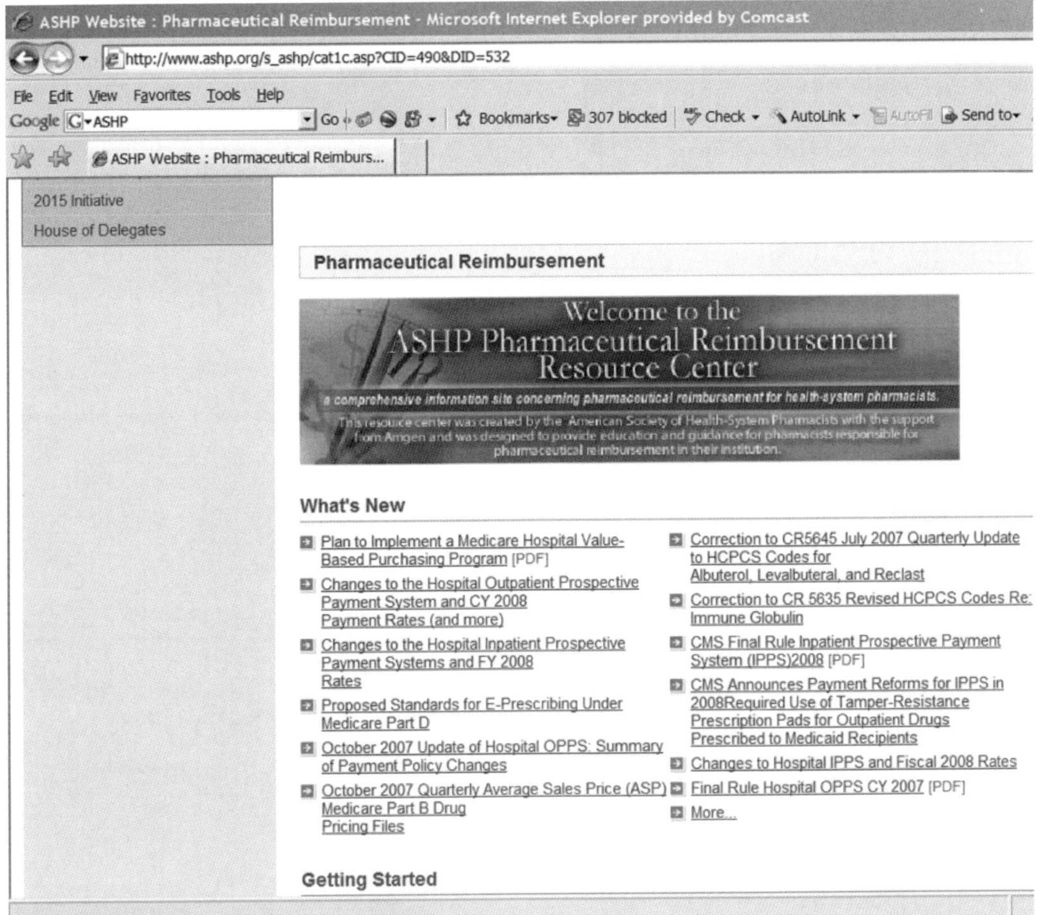

The *What's New* category contains the following information:

- Changes to the Inpatient and Outpatient Prospective Payment Systems (IPPS and OPPS)
- Proposed standards
- Quarterly Average Sales Price (ASP) data

The *Getting Started* category includes the heading "Overview for Specific Topics," which includes the following information:

- Reimbursement Building Blocks
- A Guide for Reluctant Pharmacists (A primer)
- Revenue Cycle

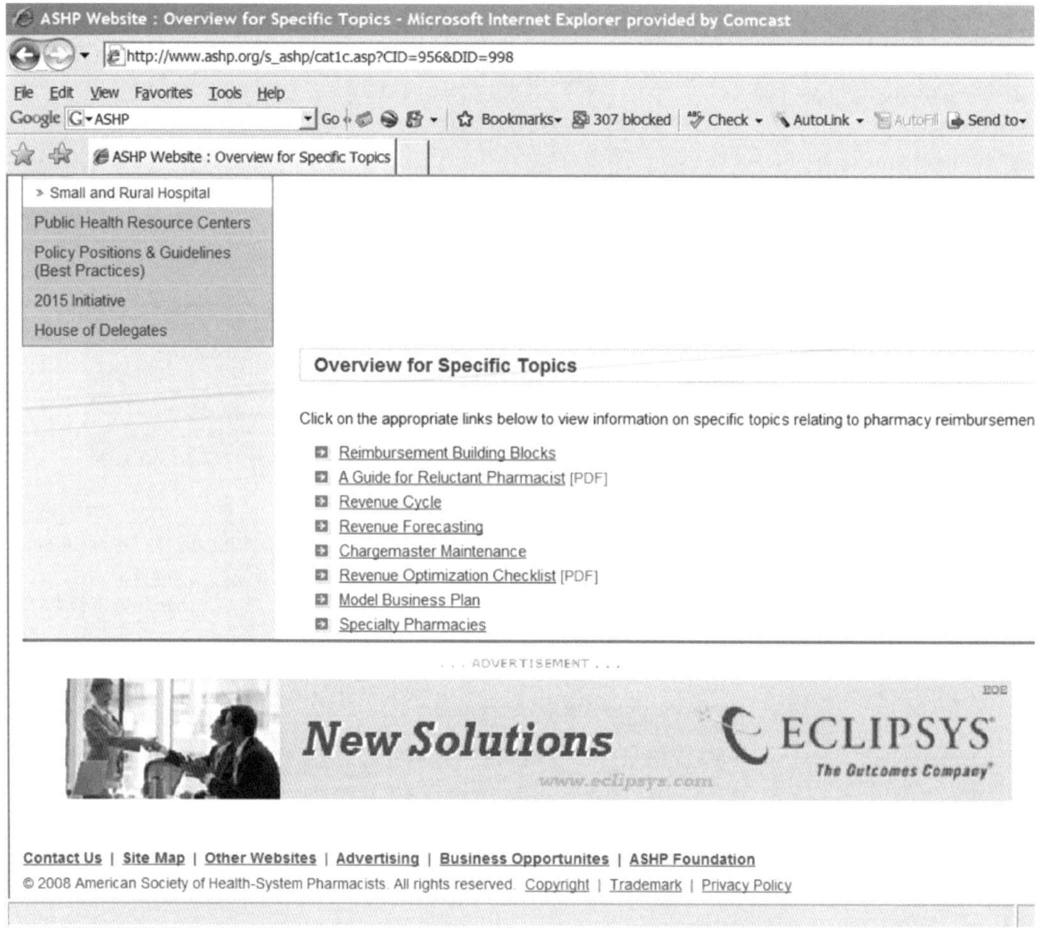

- Chargemaster Maintenance
- Revenue Optimization Checklist
- Model Business Plan
- Specialty Pharmacies

You will also find "FAQs" (Frequently Asked Questions) in this area of the website. "Strategies for Success" contains the following information:

- Essential Reimbursement Stakeholders
- Tools for Evaluating High Impact Drugs
- Reimbursement Programs
- Reimbursement Specialists

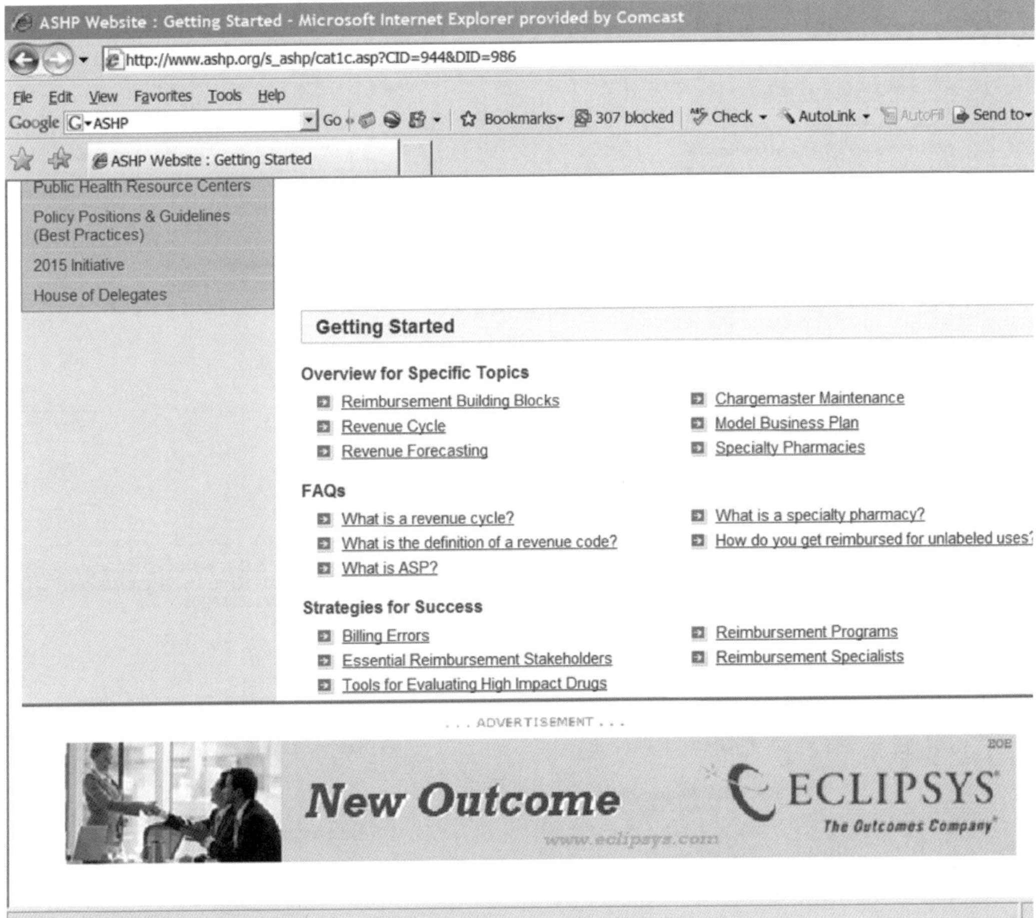

Under *Learn More*, you'll see the following headings:

- Educational Opportunities
- Articles and Publications
- Coding
- Changes in Reimbursement Rates and Rules Associated with the Medicare Prescription Drug Improvement and Modernization Act

Tools for Practice contains the following information:

- Advocacy
- CMS Resources
- Federal Register

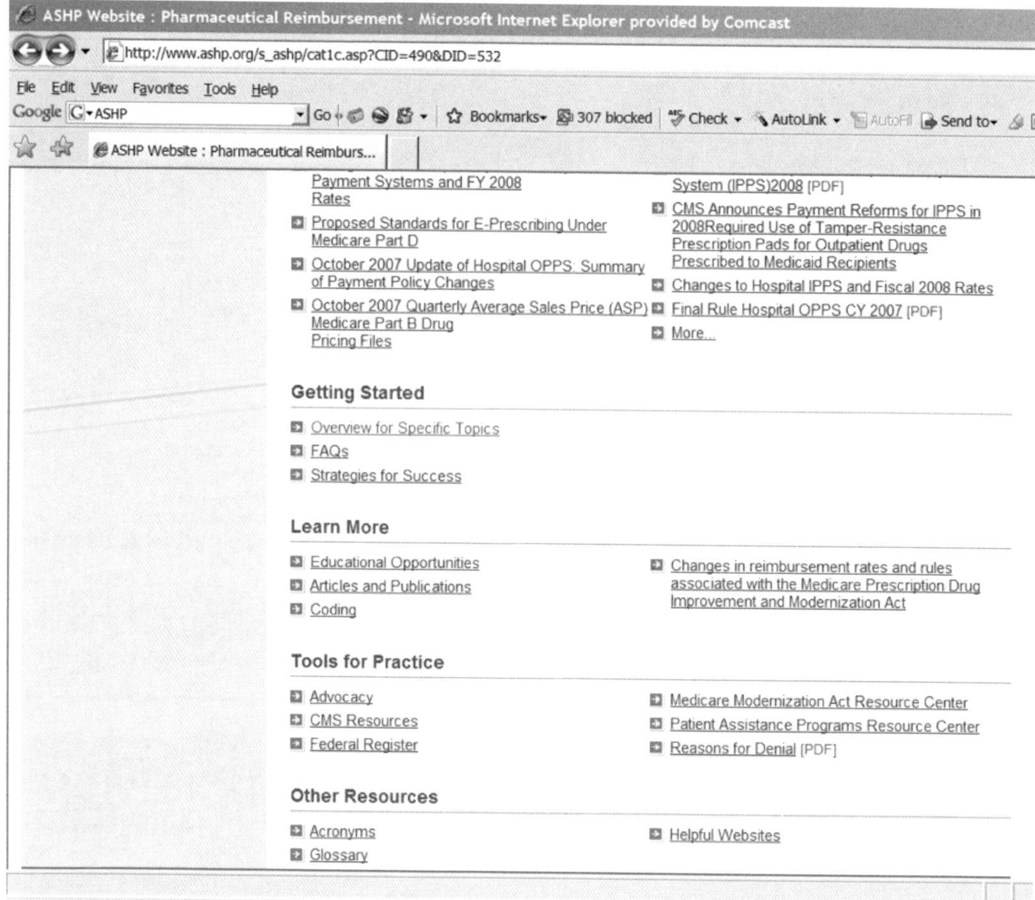

- MMA Resource Center
- PAPs Resource Center
- Reasons for Denial

And, under the heading, *Other Related Resources*, you'll find the following information:

- Acronyms
- Glossary
- Organizations
- Useful Web Sites

Whenever you need information about pharmaceutical reimbursement, ASHP's Resource Center is the place to go.

Revenue Optimization: Dollars and Sense—Are Your Revenues Optimized?

Nancy T. Nguyen
Rita Shane

Background

Optimizing revenue involves decreasing drug expenditures and maximizing reimbursement. Revenue optimization may be a more complex process than what one may have previously thought due to a multitude of factors: increase in drug expenditures as a result of new drug development, drug safety concerns, Medicare Part D drug benefit implementation, a rise in spending on biologics,[1] and the changing rules and rates for pharmaceutical reimbursement under Medicare.[2]

Description of Collaborative Effort

Due to the complexity of optimizing revenue within the pharmacy department of a health-system, the ASHP Section Advisory Group (SAG) on Financial Reimbursement identified the development of a Revenue Optimization Checklist as one of its committee goals in 2007. This collaborative effort was acknowledged as one of the tools that could be of assistance to members. It is posted on the ASHP reimbursement website and can be continually updated by any member. The checklist is organized into specific sections that prompts a "yes" or "no" response. If the response is a "yes," then that specific financial criterion is at the optimal level; if the response is a "no," then improvements can be made to either possibly increase revenue or prevent further loss of revenue by the pharmacy department.

Results

Key financial strategies for optimizing revenue primarily include reimbursement and cost avoidance and increasing revenue. Reimbursement is tied to understanding key areas within the revenue cycle, whereas cost avoidance is related to reducing expenses (for example: 340B pricing or product replacement for indigent patients).

Through the exchange of ideas and the experiences gathered by the various committee members from different institutions, a revenue optimization checklist (Table 14.1) was developed and posted on the ASHP reimbursement website in mid 2007. Categories were separated into the following and presented at various financial sessions during the Winter 2007 meeting:

- Chargemaster
- Pharmacy Systems Maintenance
- Outpatient Revenue Cycle Management
- Contracting
- 23 Hour Patients
- Charge Capture
- Other

Case Examples

Due to the variety of the categories and the large number of questions, a few key points were selected and expanded upon as described.

Case 1. Chargemaster

Are all new drugs on the formulary on the Chargemaster? Is the CMS website checked to determine if new drugs have codes assigned?

The Centers for Medicare and Medicaid Services (CMS) makes most of their changes on January 1st but updates their codes on a quarterly basis. The Chargemaster includes categories such as description, billing units, Healthcare Common Procedure Coding Systems (HCPCS) codes, revenue codes, and reimbursement rates. Accuracy of the Chargemaster is essential for appropriate billing and reimbursement. For example, some drugs are billed differently like iron sucrose (Venofer ®) or Infliximab (Remicade ®). The billing unit for iron sucrose is 1 mg, which equals 1 service unit. Therefore, when quantities greater than 1 mg of iron sucrose are given, such as 100 mg, the total amount must be billed as multiple service units. Infliximab is billed similarly; the billing unit assigned by CMS is 10 mg. If a dose of 100 mg is billed, the total billing units is 10 (for a conversion factor of 10). It is imperative that all drugs on the Chargemaster are accurate to ensure proper billing and reimbursement.

Case 2. Pharmacy Systems Maintenance

Does Pharmacy have access to financial systems to review billed charges and reimbursement, including patient and payer specific data?

Table 14.1. Revenue Optimization Checklist

Chargemaster		
Are HCPCS codes included in the Chargemaster for all drugs that have a code?	❑ Yes	❑ No
Since some drugs have both an APC and HCPCS code, is the APC included?	❑ Yes	❑ No
Are the correct revenue codes assigned to drugs?	❑ Yes	❑ No
Do all blood clotting factors have revenue code 636, HCPCS codes, and correct billing units and conversion factors?	❑ Yes	❑ No
Is there someone in pharmacy responsible for updating HCPCS codes in the Chargemaster?	❑ Yes	❑ No
Are CMS changes reviewed quarterly and is the Chargemaster updated?	❑ Yes	❑ No
Are drugs with a status indicator (SI) A, F, G, K, L coded correctly? Are they periodically updated?	❑ Yes ❑ Yes	❑ No ❑ No
Does Medicaid have medication codes that need to be included in Chargemaster?	❑ Yes	❑ No
Are the billing units and conversion factors correct? (for example: 100 mg vial of Rituxumab: billing units = 10 mg ,conversion factor = 10)	❑ Yes	❑ No
Are Medicaid changes reviewed periodically and is the Chargemaster updated to reflect any of the changes?	❑ Yes	❑ No
Are all new drugs on the formulary on the Chargemaster? Is CMS site checked to determine if new drugs have codes assigned?	❑ Yes	❑ No
Are pharmacy charge formulas for outpatient drugs periodically reviewed to ensure that charges are competitive?	❑ Yes	❑ No
Are our charge formulas taking into account price sensitive items?	❑ Yes	❑ No
Pharmacy Systems Maintenance		
Pharmacy has access to financial systems to review billed charge and reimbursement, including patient and payer specific data	❑ Yes	❑ No
Outpatient Revenue Cycle Management		
Is pharmacy a part of a revenue cycle team?	❑ Yes	❑ No
Is there a preauthorization process in place for outpatient infusion therapies and high cost injectables?	❑ Yes	❑ No
Are infusions coded accurately with respect to diagnosis and procedure? Are the codes submitted with the bill? Are administration codes included?	❑ Yes ❑ Yes ❑ Yes	❑ No ❑ No ❑ No
Is there a periodic evaluation of reimbursement for infusion therapies? By drug?	❑ Yes	❑ No
Is there a mechanism for alerting pharmacy to review drug related payment denials?	❑ Yes	❑ No
Are national and local medical review policies regarding drugs eligible for reimbursement known? Are the policies updated?	❑ Yes	❑ No
Are the proper POS (Place of Service) codes documented?	❑ Yes	❑ No
Are individual claims reviewed?	❑ Yes	❑ No
Are co-pays and/or coinsurance collected?	❑ Yes	❑ No
Is patient's payer status current and accurate?	❑ Yes	❑ No
Was claim billed to the correct payer?	❑ Yes	❑ No
Was the reimbursement received consistent with the payer specific contract?	❑ Yes	❑ No
Was revenue posted to the correct account?	❑ Yes	❑ No
Contracting		
Is the contracting department routinely notified of new expensive drug therapies that have been added to formulary?	❑ Yes	❑ No
Do expensive drugs have a "carve out" with payers for inpatients? (e.g. Factors)	❑ Yes	❑ No
Is pharmacy asked to provide input as contracts are negotiated, particularly for outpatient care?	❑ Yes	❑ No
Do contracts for outpatient care contain any language re: infusion therapies or any other medications? If yes, are there specific requirements for billing, e.g. NDC codes?	❑ Yes	❑ No
23 Hour Patients		
Are 23 hour visits being coded correctly?	❑ Yes	❑ No
Is 340B inventory being used for 23 hour pts?	❑ Yes	❑ No
Are 23 hour visits being coded as outpatient or observation, rather than as inpatients?	❑ Yes	❑ No
Charge Capture		
Is there periodic monitoring and tracking of factor patients to ensure correct and appropriate billing since there is additional Medicare reimbursement for inpatients?	❑ Yes	❑ No
Are charges being captured for medications administered in: • Diagnostic areas? • Procedural areas? • Clinics and physicians' offices?	 ❑ Yes ❑ Yes ❑ Yes	 ❑ No ❑ No ❑ No
Are audits of charges vs. purchases vs. inventory performed for top 20 drugs by cost (e.g., >$5,000/dose and by total expenditures to ensure charge capture?	❑ Yes	❑ No
Are actual payments tracked?	❑ Yes	❑ No
Other		
Is the institution getting product replacement for indigent pts?	❑ Yes	❑ No
Do you have a financial coordinator or someone from the pharmacy department to help coordinate with patient assistance programs?	❑ Yes	❑ No

At Virginia Commonwealth University Medical Center (VCUHS), pharmacists collaborate with the managed care department to review contracts [3]; contracts can potentially affect the pharmacy department because of reimbursement rules or formulas. At VCUHS, a copy of each contract on file is kept in the pharmacy department or reviewed by them semi-annually or annually to determine if renegotiations are necessary because the terms may no longer be favorable. This collaboration has led to the resolution of issues including those involving private commercial contracts. More specifically, due to the high cost of drugs, members of the pharmacy department have also collaborated with the oncology department. In general, this collaboration has led to reviews of denials and outstanding balances and has allowed the pharmacy department to ensure that reimbursement checks are received and posted to the correct accounts.

Case 3. Revenue Cycle Management

Is pharmacy a part of a revenue cycle team?

The process of revenue cycle management begins when the patient enters the system and includes all transactions that lead to revenue generation and ends with revenue collection. Since errors can occur at any point in the process, this checkpoint may involve interaction and collaboration with members of other departments within the health care system. One aspect of revenue cycle management involves pre-authorizations. For example, with the medication Infliximab, a pre-authorization is obtained for the infusion but is a pre-authorization for the drug necessary as well? It may be necessary to obtain authorizations for both. One of the last parts of the process involves claims denials. In the review of denials, pharmacists may be a good resource for understanding and resolving any issues as related to revenue recovery that will enable the resubmission of the claim since they may have a better understanding of the complete medication use process.

Case 4. Contracting

When applicable, do expensive drugs have a "carve out" with payers for inpatients?

Some private payers will not pay for some medications separately but CMS will. Blood factors are an example of this; Medicare rules for the reimbursement of blood coagulation factor products differ from other pharmaceuticals. An example was seen at Wake Forest University Baptist Medical Center in which a Medicare beneficiary was admitted for 3 months due to sustaining a head injury and required $1.4 million worth of Factor VIIa (Novoseven ®). The DRG payment, which was coded correctly, was only $100,000. Once pharmacy was made aware, they educated the billing and finance department on the separate reimbursement of Factors. They resubmitted the claim to Medicare and received additional reimbursement for the Factor drug itself.[4] Therefore it is critical that Factors and other medications that are agreed upon by private payers are billed and documented appropriately to ensure reimbursement. Also, when the opportunity arises, it may also be beneficial to focus on the most costly drugs within your health system to negotiate carve-outs with private payers.

Case 5. Charge Capture

Are audits of charges vs. purchases vs. inventory performed for top drugs as determined by cost and by total expenditures to ensure charge capture?

It is critical to look at charge capture for high cost medications; charging based on administration is an important part of revenue cycle management. At Cedars-Sinai Medical Center, we compare charges versus purchases versus inventory of some of our high cost items (by dose and by total expenditures) on a monthly basis. In late 2006, we began to notice that our purchases of thrombin were consistently higher than our charges. This was also around the same time frame that our ORs implemented a new computer system to track medications administered. In our reconciliation process, we discovered that the OR nurses were not documenting usage appropriately, which led to lost charges and therefore lost revenue. Since then, we've educated our nurses on appropriate documentation realized improvements.

Conclusion

The Revenue Optimization Checklist serves as a systematic reference for determining whether a facility has optimized all potential strategies to increase reimbursement and decrease revenue loss. The current checklist was also developed with the intention of prompting other ideas that can be further tailored to fit different health system's organizational needs. To maximize the benefits, the list must be updated to represent the current regulations and re-evaluated to ensure continuous compliance. Resources that can assist in revenue optimization include both the ASHP reimbursement website (www.ashp.org/reimburse) and the CMS website (www.cms.hhs.gov).

References

1. Hoffman JM, Shah ND, Vermeulen LC, et al. Projecting future drug expenditures – 2008. *Am J Hosp Pharm* 2008; 65:234-53.
2. Fijalka S, Fye D, Johnson PE. Current issues in pharmaceutical reimbursement. *Am J Hosp Pharm* 2008; 65 (Suppl 1):S11-26.
3. Lloyd, Laurel M. Optimizing pharmaceutical reimbursement: One institution's approach. *Am J Health-Syst Pharm* 2006; 63 (Suppl 7):S18-21.
4. Jarrett, Anne T. Understanding basic concepts and strategies for obtaining pharmaceutical reimbursement. *Am J Health-Syst Pharm* 2006; 63 (Suppl 7):S7-9.

Purchasing Strategy to Maximize Health-System Cost Savings and Improve Drug Procurement Safety

Joel A. Hennenfent
Larry J. Koesterer
Annette M. Karageanes

Background and Introduction

An epidemic of waste blights the United States healthcare delivery system.[1] Despite a large dedication of resources to healthcare in the U.S., the medical system does not deliver safe, effective, efficient, patient-centered, timely, and equitable care as recommended by the Institute of Medicine.[1-2]

One component of the high cost of healthcare is lack of efficiency in the supply chain management of medical devices, medical and non-medical supplies, and pharmaceuticals.

For example, within hospitals and health systems, many departments may purchase, and use numerous suppliers for items such as albumin, intravenous immune globulins (IVIG), Rho D immune globulins, blood factors, anesthesia gases, contrast media, nutritionals, and hemostatic agents. A purchasing strategy that utilizes preferred distributors, such as pharmacy wholesaler, medical supplies distributor, or radiology distributor, is an effective way to control costs and provide value-added benefits. This purchasing strategy leverages the lower distributor markups, provides greater visibility and review of group purchasing organization (GPO)-negotiated pricing, and increases GPO contract compliance.

Health System

Ascension Health is transforming healthcare by providing the highest quality care to all, with special attention to those who are poor and vulnerable. Ascension Health, which provided $808 million in community benefit and in care of persons who are poor last year, is the nation's largest Catholic and nonprofit health system. Our mission-focused Health Ministries consist of 106,000 associates serving in 20 states and the District of Columbia. With operating revenues of $12.3 billion, Ascension Health spent in excess of $527 million on pharmaceuticals and plasma derivatives during 2007.

Pharmacy Community

The Ascension Health Pharmacy Council guides system-wide pharmaceutical quality improvement and cost-containment initiatives for the health system. The Pharmacy Council consists of Pharmacy Directors from across the Health Ministries and System Office Pharmacy staff, including: the Senior Director of Pharmacy, Group Purchasing and Support Services; the Pharmacy Clinical Resource Specialist; the Pharmacy Contract Administrator; and a Clinical Liaison from Broadlane, Ascension Health's GPO. Pharmacy Council responsibilities include, but are not limited to, making decisions and recommendations regarding system-wide pharmacy safety, quality, and cost-containment initiatives, and sharing "best practices" for formulary and drug utilization management. In addition, one of the guiding principles of the Ascension Health Pharmacy Community is that "pharmacy practice is indivisible." That is, no element of clinical, operational, or supply chain pharmacy practice can be viewed in isolation of the other elements. All of the pharmacy practice elements work together to provide safe, high quality patient care.

Purchasing Strategy

The purchasing strategy goal is to reduce supply costs by implementing a five step process as presented in Table 15.1. When implementing this process, Ascension Health's preferred pharmacy wholesaler and blood products distributor should be used to purchase all necessary products. This will require the health system to:

- Request that these suppliers add items not currently available to ensure maximum product coverage.
- Request that all billing be managed through the pharmacy wholesaler. This consolidated billing provides a single source for reporting purchasing data.
- Request the billing be managed by the pharmacy wholesaler to ensure that purchasing data can still be provided by a single source when directly ordering from the manufacturer.
- Only utilize the medical/surgical distributor when products are not available through the preferred pharmacy wholesaler, blood products distributor or by direct order.
- Eliminate alternative "gray" market purchases to ensure patient safety, drug pedigree compliance, and reduce the risk of purchasing improperly stored or counterfeit products. Always remember, patient safety is the most important consideration when implementing each process step.

Cost Savings Analysis

A cost-savings analysis to track the on-going success of the program is critical for demonstrating value to Senior Leadership and garnering participation from departments outside pharmacy. Perform a savings analysis by comparing product usage data from two time periods. Benchmark the baseline data from the time period immediately prior to implementing the new purchasing strategy and compare this with the same time period one year later. Aggregate the data from all hospitals to develop system savings. Utilize all data from the wholesalers, distributors, manu-

Table 15.1 Five-Step Purchasing Strategy

Purchasing Strategy	
Step 1	• Utilize the health system's preferred pharmacy wholesaler, purchasing as many of the health system's needed products as possible via that route. • Request that the wholesaler stock additional pharmaceutical or non-pharmaceutical items to meet the patient needs
Step 2	• Utilize the health system's preferred blood products distributor • Purchase as many of the health system's needed products from the blood products distributor should they not be available through the pharmacy wholesaler • When possible, bill items through the health system's preferred pharmacy wholesaler • Request the blood products distributor to carry additional items in product categories to meet the patient needs
Step 3	• Utilize the manufacturer drop shipment or direct order processes • When possible, bill items through the health system's preferred pharmacy wholesaler
Step 4	• Utilize the health system's preferred medical/surgical distributors • Purchase all products from the medical/surgical distributors when they are not available from the pharmacy wholesaler, blood products distributor or manufacturer
Step 5	• Eliminate alternative "gray" market purchases o Improve patient safety o Ensure drug pedigree standard compliance o Reduce the risk of purchasing improperly stored products o Reduce risk of purchasing counterfeit products

facturers and alternative "gray" market to project the potential cost savings and anticipated changes in work volume. Develop a plan for implementing the purchasing strategy and provide appropriate staff education. After collecting the data from period two, calculate the actual cost savings and validate the strategy effectiveness.

Data Barriers

Obtaining the actual baseline data necessary for calculating cost savings may present a challenge. If the health system is not using a standardized purchasing system, it is particularly difficult to identify and capture product purchases from non-pharmacy departments. For example, items for the blood bank or dietary services may be purchased through many supply channels with minimal access to purchase history. Purchase order entry nomenclature is not often standardized and presents obstacles for compiling accurate data. In addition, multiple supply channels have varied cost structures that complicate the savings analysis compared with the new purchasing strategy, which only has two cost structures.

Multiple supply channels may utilize wholesalers or distributors with private contract agreements. When the system office is unaware of the agreement terms, it becomes hard to quantify the data. There are numerous external factors that impact the data quality and are potential barriers to gathering and quantifying data. These factors include calculating fluctuating price changes, contract changes, and drug cost inflation. New generic products, brand products, and clinical data changes impact the product mix and make utilization difficult to quantify as well. If a hospital qualifies for 340B or disproportionate share hospital (DSH) pricing or has patient mix or acuity changes, additional barriers are created. In addition, length of stay (LOS), number of admissions, and changes in facilities or services can also impact data.

Implementation Barriers

The ability to identify non-pharmacy departments that are purchasing products available through the pharmacy wholesaler and blood products distributor, and determine who should be utilizing the new purchasing strategy, presents a barrier to implementation. Introducing the purchasing strategy and obtaining acceptance of this new idea may be challenging; however, this is crucial for success. It may be difficult to get consensus among the non-pharmacy departments to a joint strategy, utilizing the new purchasing model, and developing a policy. Options to overcoming these barriers include using the Department of Pharmacy Services to order and distribute products to the other departments or having non-pharmacy departments establish an account with the appropriate wholesaler or blood products distributor. The latter alternative allows departments to order and receive products directly from the wholesaler and not involve pharmacy in the process.

Additional Benefits

Implementing this strategy standardizes the supply chain process and improves distribution efficiency. Departments using this strategy will yield improvements in purchasing, billing, budgeting, and product distribution. By purchasing products through the preferred pharmacy wholesaler and blood products distributor, the number of systems with purchasing history decreases, and the accuracy and consistency of data improves. With improved access to quality data, the ability to monitor utilization and identify trends and cost savings initiatives also improves. Increased data accuracy allows Health Ministries to contract products more effectively and leverage opportunities.

Minimizing distribution channels allows the ordering departments to improve inventory management and ensure the availability of appropriate products to meet patient satisfaction. Inventory turns are improved and product waste is minimized as a result of better control over expiration dates. With fewer distribution channels, the product return process is simplified. The process for returning unused or expired products is easier and has more value in a health system's preferred medication returns reverse distribution system. Increased revenue can be captured by evaluating cost structures and standardizing to the highest charge formula where appropriate. Moreover, there are opportunities to improve patient safety in addition to the financial benefits.

Conclusions

Implementation of this purchasing strategy has the potential to significantly reduce supply costs. The purchasing strategy is applicable for all products available through the pharmacy wholesaler and blood products distributor. The largest cost saving is generated by identifying products non-pharmacy departments are purchasing from medical/surgical or alternative "gray" market distributors that are available from the pharmacy wholesaler or blood products distributor at a better value. Components of the purchasing strategy should be incorporated into the department and hospital performance scorecard to successfully achieve strategy compliance (eg, develop a metric that 100% of albumin purchases must be obtained from the preferred blood products distributor). In addition, align the administrative performance bonus to the compliance performance metric. With effective compliance, monitoring, communication, and incentives, the organization will maximize cost savings and improve drug procurement safety.

References

1. Bush RW. Reducing waste in US health care systems. *JAMA* 2007; 297(8):871-4.
2. Institute of Medicine (IOM). Crossing the quality chasm: the IOM health care quality initiative. Available at http://www.iom.edu/CMS/8089.aspx. Accessed May 14, 2008.

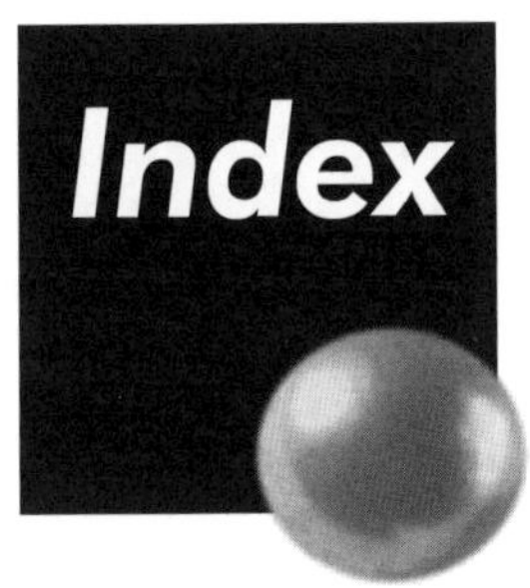
Index

U

V